DETOX ME JUICY

PRAISE FOR PETRA'S BOOKS

"I love this book! I would recommend this book to anyone and everyone. It is a total life-changer! We must choose joy every day and this book gives us the tools we need to be successful. This experience has definitely motivated my mind and inspired my heart. I truly needed this book to capture myself."

- Sylva, Chili & Chocolate Blogger, Czech

"I have never come across a book written with so much enthusiasm, strong knowing of the power of CHOICE and how to create that in your life! Louise Hay started the affirmation movement but this book is designed in a way so that when you read it you are already saying the affirmations much less learning how to act as if they were and are already true. It is the kind of book I have on coffee table by bed so I can read a chapter in 5-10 minutes if feeling blue or unsure about life, reminding myself who I really am and all I can BE on this planet! Love it!"

-Margaret, Naturopathic Doctor, USA

"I love myself so much more after reading this book. As soon as I finished it, I started reading it again. It has given me so much personal power and self worth. I am so grateful I bought this book and met Petra in person."

- Yorgi, Yoga Geek, Germany

"I have just finished your book and wanted to tell you how grateful I was to have crossed your way. Your words were awakening ideas that I already know somehow but so good to hear it this way. They have been nourishing my thoughts and heart lately. Thank you."

- Aline, Australia

"I found your book '5 Things I Love About You' and it was the best gift I could find before hosting my first yoga retreat. You described in beautiful words what I wanted to share with my yoga tribe. A few days into my retreat, I found another book of yours, 'I Am Amazing' and had to buy it immediately. Some of my students followed me and bought the book too. I just finished reading it and I am beyond grateful that I found it. You really inspire me and you write about so many things I totally believe in! Thank you for sharing your awesomeness with this world. I love learning more from you!"

- Audrey, Yoga Teacher, Austria

"Thank you for shining your AWESOMENESS, your AMAZINGNESS and your ROCKSTAR attitude into the words of this book! It was life-changing for me at a time when I truly felt the world was not on my side. I keep this book with me all the time as it is my bible, my life saver, my life changer and my life up-leveler. Thank you and stay cool my sista!!"

- Lizzy, Champion Ski Racer, Canada

"Thank you for the positive impact you have had on my life. I'm relishing a lot of fabulous thoughts and notions from all kinds of sources now, and it all started with your book, so I'm really grateful. This morning, I got up to see the sun rise over the sea and then went for a run, soaking up all the beautiful nature along the way. Life is good and I can really appreciate it due to your book!"

- Johanna, Spain

"A feel-good read, bursting with energy and positivity. This book has played an important part in my journey of self-discovery and happiness for which I am really grateful."

- Scott, Head Chief Animation School, Canada

"I've finished your book! Loved it and was sad to finish it as I so enjoyed reading it. Am recommending it to some friends I know will cherish it too. I've started a journal and have always practiced gratitude but now am listing 10 things when I wake up. So much in your book I had a huge connection with. Thank you from my heart. Your book came to me at exactly the right time and as you so rightly said, there are no coincidences."

- Rachel, Pilates Personal Trainer, Spain

"I can tell this book is written by a woman who understands the importance of self-care through intense personal experience. She has helped me and my friends change the way we see ourselves. She is amazing and I now carry Petra's mantra, 'Unfold your wings and fly'. I can't wait for the newest book to arrive."

- Denise, Hotel Owner, Indonesia

"Very uplifting book that definitely raised my vibration! This book and the author are so positive. Anyone who is struggling with self-love and self-compassion would find this book useful. I highly recommend giving it a try."

- Rebecca, Pro Surfer, Hawaii

"Petra, you truly radiate light and love and all that is good in the world. You ARE amazing, thanks for being that beacon of hope and swagger, reminding us that we are truly special. Love your juicy cleansing and this just makes me want even MORE from you. Thank you, You ROCK!"

- Pat, Life & Business Coach, New York

"A positive and powerful way to live! This book is my bible and one to keep close. So happy I read it."

- Ginger, Movie Script Supervisor, Canada

"This book is amazing!!!! When I look in the mirror and say the title out loud, I feel the truth resonating from the top of my head to the bottom of my feet. My personal doubts slowly disappeared upon reading this book and I really am able to do anything I ever wanted to do. Thank you Petra for sharing your amazing truth and helping wake the world up and heal all of our wounded hearts. I am ready to love myself more and I am so happy I read this book."

- Rick, Hypnotherapist & Spiritual Alchemist, Arizona

"This book was bought as a gift and I loved it! So many things Petra writes resonates with me on a deep level. Upon reading it, I learned so much, I had so many ideas, I felt so many emotions and it really opened me up. This was a life changing book for me and will always be so special."

- Nedi, Morning News Producer, Africa

"Fantastic book, especially whenever I need a positive charge! Petra's words literally seethe right off the page and I cannot help but smile. I believe in myself more and more as I read the words like mantras. Easy to read, down-to-earth and authentic! I highly recommended it!"

- Pamela, Coffee Barista, Amsterdam

"Petra is an amazing being. She is always uplifting, great sense of humor, speaks straight to the point and is fantastic chef! She is courageous and dedicated to her mission to heal the world and empower the women. Petra walks her talk. This book is beautiful, funny and authentic."

- Mariola, Yogini & Model, Hawaii

DETOX
ME
JUICY

The 7 Day Juicy Food Cleanse To Lose Weight, Youthen
& Heal Your Body Of Everything

PETRA EATJUICY
Green Smoothie Gangster

DETOX ME JUICY

ISBN 9781983274701

Cover design by Petra EatJuicy & Adityah Kasim
Book Design by Petra EatJuicy & Adityah Kasim

Visit me on the web!
www.EatJuicy.com
www.GreenSmoothieGangster.com

Tell me how you liked the book!
www.Facebook.com/PetraEatJuicy

First Edition: 2018

Thank you for buying this book.

It is my intention that after reading it, you are more
confident and ready to cleanse your body
and know you can do it.

You will feel energized, lighter, clearer, more grounded
and more in love with yourself.

Free video lessons & recipes at

www.EatJuicy.com
www.GreenSmoothieGangster.com

www.Facebook.com/PetraEatJuicy
www.Youtube.com/PetraEatJuicy
www.Instagram.com/PetraEatJuicy

> "LET FOOD BE YOUR MEDICINE &
> MEDICINE BE YOUR FOOD"

Hippocrates – Father of Medicine
Oath sworn by ALL Western medical doctors, Yet NOT used by MOST

Therefore....

> "TAKE YOUR HEALTH INTO YOUR HANDS.
> UNDERSTAND YOUR BODY AND HOW IT WORKS. KNOWLEDGE IS POWER.
> FLUSH YOUR TOXINS OUT WITH LIQUIDS & LEARN TO ADORE YOURSELF.
> YOUR BODY IS A SELF HEALING MACHINE,
> ALL YOU HAVE TO DO IS GET OUT OF THE WAY &
> LET THE HEALING TAKE PLACE"

Petra EatJuicy – Cleanse & Detox Expert

CONTENTS

YOU ARE POWERFUL

YOU ARE AMAZING

YOU ARE STRONG

YOU ARE BRAVE

YOU ARE REALLY, REALLY SMART

YOU ARE LOVEABLE

YOU ARE SO LOVED

YOU ARE LOVED BY THE UNIVERSE

YOU ARE LOVED BY EVERYONE

YOU ARE REALLY SPECIAL

YOU ARE EXCEPTIONAL

YOU ARE EXTRAORDINARY

YOU ARE CLEVER

YOU ARE ENOUGH

YOU ARE ENOUGH

- - ♡ - -

A LOVE NOTE FROM PETRA

MY MOM WAS DIAGNOSED WITH CANCER, 14 years ago and died within 3 months. During those 3 months I researched all the ways we could heal her naturally. Unfortunately at the time, my knowledge was too little and our time was too short. I also didn't fully understand how the body worked, that it actually naturally heals itself and that the body does have the power to heal from ALL sickness.

Had I known back then, what I know now and what is written in this book, I believe with all my being that my mom would have a massive chance at recovery. Of course, she herself would have to believe in her OWN ability to self heal and then allow her body to do the work. No pill, doctor or procedure can heal us, it is our own body's natural self healing mechanism and our internal belief system that actually heals us. We have to purify the body to help it function optimally as it is designed to do. We and our body intelligence are very powerful.

My mom's death is a terrible tragic devastating event in my life that still brings tears to my eyes. Over time I had to find a positive reasoning to her death and now know it launched me on the trajectory to learn everything I can about disease prevention, self healing, full life empowerment and radical self love. I have accumulated all this knowledge so I may share it with all of you, so your life can be more extraordinary. I have studied with the best teachers and teach all over the world, inspiring people on their own life transformations.

It is my intent with this book, that you know you are more powerful than you have been lead to believe and that you realize your body can fully repair itself if given the right space, right amount of time and the right form of cleaning. Let's face it, in order for you to be healthy and happy, YOU HAVE to have a body that works for you. This book is one tool for you to heal your body, rejuvenate your life and step into your full power as a super human on this planet.

Maybe you have been curious about eating healthier, doing a JUICY cleanse or starting to make more powerful food choices in your life but have not known where to start. In this book, I guide you on cleansing your body and giving your digestive system a break. Our body is always doing 1 of 2 things, it is either digesting our food or it is healing our body. If we are constantly eating heavy hard to digest food, then our body is always working hard at digesting and has no time for our healing. With the increase of toxins in our food, our water and our air, our body gets over burdened and stops being able to function properly.

The toxins build up in our cells, in our blood and in our lymphatic fluid. The body gets poisoned, tired and moves into dis-ease. Maybe your body is already giving you small signals like head aches, ear aches, body aches, eczema or skin rashes? Are you listening and acting naturally to heal from the inside out? Or are you using pharmaceutical drugs or steroid creams to mask your symptoms thinking that if they go away, you are healed? All our external symptoms are an indication of an imbalance inside of us and unless we address the inside, then the imbalance will show up somewhere else in our body and perhaps next time, it will show up bigger.

We are energetic beings. We are made up of energy. We are energy inside a skin bag and have enough voltage to light a 15 watt light bulb. If our energy stops properly flowing, if we don't know how to recharge our system or if something inside us short circuits our energy, then dis-ease will set in.

It is my intention that you take time to heal, cleanse and purify your body to prevent dis-ease from ever coming to get you. If you already have dis-ease, then it is my intention that you know (with your whole heart and soul) that YOU CAN heal it.

Dis-ease is not something that comes to attack us like a big monster as the medical system would have us believe. It is co-created inside our body by our thoughts, our beliefs, the environments and the fuel we put inside our body.

So how do we get healthy? Simple. We cleanse the body of toxins and help move the energy inside our body to flow once more.

The following chapters will guide you on doing a JUICY food cleanse from the comfort of your home. You don't have to drink only juices to cleanse, I will teach you various ways of cleansing and you can feel into which method is right for you. If you have a sickness or you want to create healing in your body quickly, then please do a green juice or water cleanse to expedite your process. Cut out sugar completely and alkaline your body with greens as fast as possible. You are worth it and your life may depend on it.

For most of us, the thought of letting go of food or not chewing is extremely frightening and we feel it doesn't seem doable. For years I have been leading juice detox cleanses all over the world in person and online I promise, you won't starve, feel weak or be unable to do this. On the contrary, the amount of nutrition you receive from raw juices and raw food, will give your body so much life force and vitamins that you will feel amazing and energized.

If you want to lose weight, heal your gut, get rid of constipation, have beautiful skin, feel energized or heal sickness in your body, then doing a JUICY food cleanse is the first step.

Yes, it takes bravery to make a change and I know you can do this. The scariest thing is to stop eating. Eating is a habit. Even when we are not hungry, we eat out of habit. So the first few days of doing any cleanse, is about breaking habits.

Most of the time, we also eat for emotional support. Food makes us feel safe and comfortable. So stopping eating food can bring up a lot of emotions. This is good. Issues live in our tissues, so doing a cleanse will also help us release old stored up emotions that may be causing us harm.

I am super proud of you. I have got you by the hand and I am here to support and guide you. You are a powerful magical divine miraculous human creature on this planet and you deserve to feel vibrant healthy energized and thriving into your old age. Please take your health into your own hands. You are totally worth it.

With love, gratitude and aloha
Petra

GO FOR IT!

READ THIS TO YOURSELF AS YOUR NEW MANTRA:

I AM POWERFUL

I AM AMAZING

I AM STRONG

I AM BRAVE

I AM LOVEABLE

I AM LOVED

I AM ENOUGH

I LOVE MY BODY

I HEAL MY BODY

I TAKE CARE OF MY BODY

MY BODY LOVES ME

MY BODY IS ALWAYS HEALING ME

MY BODY IS WORKING 24 / 7 TO MAKE ME HEALTHY

I AM GRATEFUL FOR MY BEAUTIFUL STRONG BODY

I FEED IT THE BEST FUEL POSSIBLE

I THINK THE KINDEST MOST UPLIFTING THOUGHTS

I DRINK LOTS OF LIQUIDS

I FLUSH MY TOXINS OUT

I RELEASE WHAT IS NO LONGER SERVING ME

I RELEASE THE PHYSICAL

I RELEASE THE EMOTIONAL

I RELEASE ALL MY OLD BAGGAGE

I FLUSH ALL MY CRAP OUT

I let go
I let go
I let go
I receive vibrant health
I receive joy, happiness & bliss
I love myself
I love my body
I take care of myself
I am worth it
You are Brave
Amazing Powerful
&
Totally in control of your life

I have said YES
To taking my health
Into my hands

I have waited Long enough
To feel Healthy
Energized
&
Vibrant

I got this

It is my
Birthright To feel Amazing

MY BODY'S ABILITY TO HEAL IS
MORE POWERFUL THAN ANYONE HAS
LED ME TO BELIEVE

- - ♡ - -

LET'S USE
I AM

From this point on...the way you read this book will change. No longer will you be reading it as me writing and guiding you, now you will read it as YOU guiding YOU using the words I AM.

Reading from the YOU perspective as most books are written, might not penetrate into your consciousness and your mind might glaze over. Reading this book, using I AM will remind you that this is YOUR life, YOUR reality and YOU have choice on how it is created.

I AM are the 2 most powerful words in our vocabulary, we create our reality by the "spell" of words we weave. We can declare anything about our life and ourselves. Speaking from the I AM perspective is the gateway. I am smart or I am dumb, you get to choose your reality based on the words you use. So from now on, I will guide you subtly and vicariously through you to help reprogram your subconscious mind for ultimate empowerment and superhuman health. This book is your own personal cleansing guide. Let the information and love in. You are worth it. Time to I AM it.....

EVERY BITE I TAKE IS
EITHER HEALING ME
OR SLOWLY KILLING ME

FOOD IS MY BODY'S FUEL
OR MY POISON

- - ♡ - -

CHAPTER 1

START HERE!

WELCOME TO MY JUICY FOOD CLEANSE overview chapter...

I AM AMAZING and I AM super proud of me! Awesome Job!

Doing this JUICY food cleanse will help me unleash the natural healing power of my body. It will help me get rid of years of built up toxins. Toxins get built up in my body through the food I eat, the air I breathe, the environments I put myself in and the stress, grief and sadness I have accumulated over the years. Eating JUICY food floods my system with powerful nutrients, antioxidants and massive hydration. It may be the first step toward a long-lasting JUICY lifestyle or a healthy weight loss 7 + day regimen. Drinking JUICY will help kick start my system, activate the healing powers within, retrain my taste buds and allow me to witness the emotional connections I have to food. I will use this JUICY cleanse to release sickness out of my body and prevent it from ever coming back. If my body is out of balance in some way, then doing a JUICY food cleanse will help me get back into alignment within myself.

WHY A JUICY FOOD CLEANSE WORKS...

Dis-ease means the body is out of ease and wants to get back to its natural rhythm. In an effort to help me heal, my body will create a big red flag for me called dis-ease so I can finally see it and do something about it. In all moments of the day, my body is healing me and working for my greatest self expression on this planet. Without me having to do anything, my body is growing my hair, my fingernails and breathing me automatically. If my body gets too tired or too toxic, then it goes into dis-ease. During dis-ease, my body is trying to get rid of the huge amount of waste matter that has accumulated in my body due to my not so healthy lifestyle. Toxins get stuck in my system and ruin the normal actions of my body. The body works really hard 24/7 to get rid of these toxins, but sometimes there are too many and my body can no longer heal me.

So it needs my help. My body needs me to stop the toxic intake both physical and mental, and to start flushing with liquids, raw fruit and vegetable fiber power. My body wants me to cleanse and is so happy I am on its side. Once I cleanse my body, it can start working properly again and helping me live the most amazing life ever. I am totally worth it. I take my health into my hands starting right now.

When I stop eating solid food for several days and start eating JUICY food, then my body gets a break. My body is either healing me or digesting my food. If I am eating all the time and eating food that is hard for my body to break down, then my body is always working on digesting and has no time for my healing. When I begin eating juices, liquids and JUICY food, then my body gets a break from digesting and can focus on my healing.

It's quite a simple process for my ultimate healing. I just have to help my body already do what it was designed to do. HEAL ME!!!

The ideal length of my JUICY flushing cleanse is 7 + days. Of course my body will be happy at any level of cleansing I do, but if I want to really jump start my immune system and reboot my system then 7 or more days is ideal.

MY NEW PRE CLEANSE STARTING DIET...

Upholding a healthy, light diet at least 3 days before my JUICY food cleanse will ease the hunger cravings during my cleansing process. I eat LOTS of organic fresh fruits, vegetables, lentils, beans, seeds, nuts and whole grains like rice, quinoa and buckwheat. I drink LOTS of water to start the flushing process. I avoid alcohol, caffeine, sugar, processed foods, dairy, meat and gluten or greatly reduce it. I eat as much raw food as possible and start drinking a morning green smoothie. My morning green smoothie will be the easiest way to ease into my healthier lifestyle. I cut out all the processed, chemical and fast food take out. I start reading ingredients and becoming more aware of what I put into my body.

I will love how I feel so much that this pre cleanse diet will be the introduction to my new JUICY lifestyle that I will continue for the rest of my life. I will ease myself into cleansing, healing and detoxing and start falling in love with how my body feels.

Prepping with a healthier diet for a few days or few weeks prior is the ideal way to begin a cleansing journey YET I might have to jump right into a juice or water detox. If I am sick, need to boost my immune system FAST or am just ready to change my life then I JUST START JUICING! This is my body and my life, only I know intuitively what is best for me. I will be ok and my body will quickly support my healing and flushing process.

SETTING MY INTENTION...

I set an intention of transformation for my JUICY food cleanse. An intention is a commitment to changing a part of my life that is no longer serving me. What relationships, illnesses and thought patterns do I want to heal through my JUICY cleansing? How will I know if my JUICY cleanse is a success? I will fill in the JUICY questionnaire in this book to reveal the intention for my JUICY cleanse and ultimately the intention for my life.

I don't need a JUICY cleanse to let something go in my life that is no longer serving me, yet having the physical structure of a cleanse gives me a container to release in a more focused way. Doing a cleanse is never just about drinking juices or eating healthier food, it is always about letting go what is no longer serving me in my life and replacing it with more positive higher vibration actions and thoughts.

I take time to think about my life, my habits, my resentments, my anger, my issues, my pain and my suffering. I choose to release these harmful things out of my life and my body starting now.

I am an emotional, spiritual and energetic being along with being a physical human. I have to create whole body healing in order to thrive on this planet and I must see myself as a whole eco system that is intricately connected to everything and everyone. The medical system would have me believe that I am just a physical body and cut out of me anything that is broken. Yet everything works with everything, so I have to heal my entire system in order to be thriving.

I am not just a body that needs a cream to fix a rash. I am cosmic energy that is creating the rash from an emotional, spiritual or energetic place and I have to be willing to look at ALL of myself in order to fully heal.

MY NEW JUICY FOOD CLEANSE DIET...

Over my 7 + days, I will drink as many juices, smoothies, water, teas, soups and other liquids as possible. I will allow my body to do as little digesting as possible. I may choose to drink 100% juices and liquids which will be the most effective in jump starting my system. If I get hungry, I can add in juicy fruit, salads or quinoa. I avoid adding in too much cooked food as this will slow down my cleansing process and I definitely will stay away from processed food. I am cleansing and I am going for it, so I will make this cleanse effective.

The first few days of my cleanse might be the hardest as letting go of food is an emotional process. My body might be telling me it is hungry, that it can't survive without food or that I cannot continue. I don't let my brain or ego win. Once I let go of the pattern of needing to chew every few hours, as I have been doing for years, and replace it with eating liquids, I will see that I am actually not hungry at all.

I might feel achy, have flu like symptoms, get a head ache or feel a bit nauseous during my first few days. I am ok. I am safe. I don't stop because I think this cleanse is harming me in some way. My body is actually healing. My cells have been storing toxins and hiding them from the rest of my body as a form of protection, for years. Once my cells get the signal that I am cleaning house, they will slowly start to release my toxins into my blood stream and lymphatic fluid, so I can flush them out.

If I started cleaning a very dirty house full of garbage and recycling, my first few days in the house would make me feel sick too due to the stink and rot. Eventually as I cleaned, took the garbage out and opened up windows, my house would start feeling amazing. This is the same process I am doing by cleansing my body. My body is my skin bag house I am living in.

During my JUICY cleanse, I drink lots of liquids. I drink them as often as I need to feel satiated and energized. Ideally I have a glass of something liquid every half hour or hour. My body will adjust quickly to my new diet and I will feel surprisingly full and energized. As I start my cleanse, I will drink more liquids and drink them more often. Then as I progress in my cleanse, I might find that I feel too full to have another juice. I listen to my body. The easiest way to ensure success in my cleanse is to be organized with my liquid food supply on hand. If I get hungry and don't have a juice to grab, it is much easier for me to stray off my cleanse and cheat. So I set myself up for success and have liquid food available at all times.

I remember my body is always doing 2 functions: digesting my food or healing my body. When I give my body a break from digesting food, then my body spends all of its time on my healing. So the longer I give my body a break from eating, the longer my body works on my healing.

Ideally I do my cleanse for 7 or more days. A 1 day cleanse is great too, yet the real effects are felt after 5 + days. It usually takes the first 3 days for my body to adjust to not eating solid food. So usually by day 3, my body starts to feel energized and really good. I incorporate juicy fruit, salads or raw soups to start or throughout, if I need it.

There are no rules. Any kind of cleanse I do is amazing for my body and my body will LOVE ME. The main purpose is to give my body a break from digesting so I have a healthier body and more energized lifestyle.

Eliminating unhealthy food for a week is also a cleanse. So is eliminating gluten or dairy or meat, stopping stress and toxic thoughts. I get to choose how I want to cleanse my body. The main point of this book is to encourage me to do SOME KIND of cleanse, so I feel lighter, happier, healthier and more alive. How I get there is up to me.

I could also transition my cleanse, to drinking water only and this is the fastest way for my body to go into ketosis mode. In ketosis all my cells begin regeneration and my immune system begins to rebuild. It usually takes 72 or more hours with no sugar in my system for my body to go into ketosis. Water fasting is safe as my body can live without food. If I plan to do a water cleanse, then I drink smoothies and juices for a few days prior, then transition to water or coconut water only. It will make my transition a lot easier and ensure my success. I might feel more tired and sensitive on a water cleanse. This is because my body is not receiving any sugars, vitamins or nutrients and starts going through a very internal process. This can take up a lot of my body's energy.

If I feel crappy in the beginning of my cleanse or during, it is an indication that my body has a lot of toxins living in it. As I give my body the signals that we are cleansing, my cells open up and begin releasing the locked away toxins they were protecting me from. So it is better I feel crappy for a few days in order to feel amazing for the rest of my life. I promise myself I won't stop my JUICY cleanse even if I feel crappy. I promise to honor my higher guidance and my internal voice that might ask me to stop or act more gentle with myself. I eat light food and keep juicing, knowing I will feel really good very soon as the toxins leave my body.

MY APPROXIMATE DRINKING SCHEDULE...

I drink my JUICY liquids in 30 min or 1 hour or 2 hour increments. It will be an easier transition for me and an easier cleansing experience, if I drink more often and always have juice or a yummy liquid drink on hand at all times. I set my phone alarm to remind me to drink my liquids. I continue drinking liquids on lightly structured schedule to ensure success. I avoid starving myself and eliminate the possibility of me cheating by grabbing the closest thing near by. I follow this timetable example of Liquid Juices / Smoothies to ensure success. I add in water, herbal teas, coconut water and super food cleansers for additional hydration and cleansing.

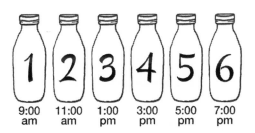

| 1 | 2 | 3 | 4 | 5 | 6 |
| 9:00 am | 11:00 am | 1:00 pm | 3:00 pm | 5:00 pm | 7:00 pm |

MY DAILY EXERCISE...

During my JUICY cleanse, I will explore doing lighter exercise, such as walks, yoga and stretching. My energy levels will change as I cleanse and I pay attention to what my body needs before exercising. I might even feel a little lightheaded if my body starts missing the sugar intake. I am ok. I take it easy. I get up slowly. I might also feel the need to stay very active, run and go to the gym for the first few days of my JUICY cleanse and I promise to be gentle with myself. I recognize that my body is healing and it needs to rest, which is an important part of the healing process. My body heals when it is resting and sleeping. I give myself rest and I take lots of power naps during my JUICY cleanse. It is totally acceptable to have a power siesta every day, as my body will use this time for regeneration. I will set my alarm for 22 or 44 min and close my eyes. I will give myself time to rest and I may also fall asleep. Sleep and rest are super healing for my body.

MY DAILY ACTIVITIES & HOW TO SPEND MY TIME...

Introspective activities such as writing in my journal, meditating, walking in nature, listening to music and dancing in my living room are incredibly healing during my JUICY cleanse (and the rest of my life). I avoid places with loud noise and a lot of activity. I might be more sensitive to energies during my JUICY food cleanse. I make a lot of free time to take care of myself. I get massages and healing work to expedite my cleansing process. I move my body in dance and yoga so the toxins can get flushed out faster. I sit in dry, wet or infrared saunas. I remember my cleanse will bring up old stored emotions and pains inside my body if I allow myself. I give myself the time and space to heal myself. I make time for ME during this cleanse. I allow myself to dig deep into myself, into my fears, wounds, pain, hopes, dreams and personality traits. I am willing to look at myself and give myself permission to question all my actions. I allow time during this cleanse to deepen the connection I have with myself and become more in love with myself in every minute.

I can also cleanse and go to work every day. I can bring juices with me, make smoothies at work or eat juicy fruit. I reduce the long work hours and give myself my evenings for rest and regeneration. I prep my juices and liquid food ahead of time daily. I create very successful cleanse even with a full calendar of activities and daily work.

MY POST CLEANSE DIET...

After I finish my 7 + day JUICY cleanse, I will ease into eating food with more awareness. I avoid heavy complicated meals as they might make me feel sick since my body is not used to this level of digesting. I ease my way into eating gently. Same as the pre cleanse diet, I add in fruits, greens, veggies, gluten free grains and lots of water. I slowly add in solid food and avoid processed food. Ideally this cleanse will ignite a healthier lifestyle desire in me and I continue the body healing process for the rest of my life by eating healthy. I break my cleanse with a green smoothie, giant fruit salad, quinoa, rice, gluten free pasta, salad or soup.

A LOVE NOTE FROM PETRA: One of my favorite things to eat to break my cleanses is quality raw chocolate and juicy fresh fruit. Yum! I also love eating plain curry sauce (no vegetables) or a vegetable broth poured over organic rice or quinoa. I avoid the cooked vegetables and just have hot plain broth. The warmth and simplicity of the food, makes my tummy feel great after cleansing. Plain cooked potatoes or quinoa with some good quality salt and olive oil are another favorite of mine. Something solid but simple always makes me feel good.

- - ♥ - -

I ELIMINATE THE NOT SO GOOD FOR ME STUFF...

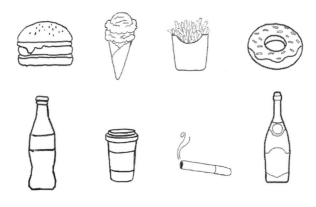

I DRINK JUICY & ADD IN THE GOOD FOR ME STUFF...

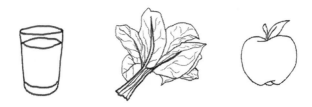

MY BODY IS ALWAYS DOING
ONE OF TWO THINGS
EITHER DIGESTING MY FOOD
OR
HEALING MY BODY

- - ♡ - -

CHAPTER 2

WHY JUICY CLEANSING?

THE PURPOSE OF THIS CLEANSE IS TO FLUSH out my system, give my digestion a break, help my body heal itself and boost my immune system. The bonus benefits will be, I lose weight, get rid of my excess fecal matter, heal my gut, heal my constipation, have glowing skin, eliminate skin issues, have tons more energy, reboot my system and put me on a healthier path fast.

My digestive system is one long tube. Food enters the top of the tube via my mouth and exits out the bottom of the tube via my bum. Food swirls through this super long bendy tube and ideally comes out the other end. Yet most of us have a dirty internal tube, old rotting food is tucked away in every bend and old caked on fecal matter is polluting our systems. Lots of mucous and plaque build up on the walls of our digestive tracks for protection from the crap we eat. In order to properly absorb nutrients and to feel healthy, we have to flush out our tube. By cleansing with JUICY liquids from both ends of the tube, we flush the garbage out. Like hair caught in my bathroom drain, I need to add cleanser along with lots of water to open up the passageways again.

In this book, I am guided to try many cleanse level options. The cleanse level I choose is up to me depending on the results I wish to attain. I choose the level that feels good for me and I am willing to stretch myself out of my comfort zone.

Whatever cleansing level I choose, I start with the pre cleanse diet to ease myself into my cleansing process. The pre cleanse diet can last a few days or a few weeks prior and it will give me many cleansing benefits. Eating clean, raw and fresh food will help me release toxins, help me lose weight and give me tons of energy.

I use this book as a guide and then listen to my own body for the wisdom. I will also watch when the ego tries to play tricks on me and talk me out of my cleansing, because it is too afraid to let go of my crap, physically and mentally.

Sometimes I have a hard time letting go of my crap. Letting go of the bullshit I have been telling myself all these years and the bullshit I continue carrying around because without it, who would I be? I now listen to that trickster inner voice that will tell me, "I don't need to cleanse. I am cleansed enough. Cleansing is for hippies. Cleansing is dangerous and I have absolutely zero crap inside my body to cleanse anyway".

If I have a belly or a lot of extra pudge around my mid section, it is not made from beer as I might be proudly convinced. It is actually an enlarged and inflamed colon. If my colon has fecal matter inside that I am not releasing fast enough, my colon organ will stretch to store all the extra crap and become much bigger. If my diet is not very healthy, then my body is acidic and my colon is inflamed and puffy. If I have been eating food that has agitated or inflamed my system, then my gut and colon are not happy.

My colon is the king to my entire system and the gut is my queen. If they are not healthy then the toxic sludge inside will affect all other parts of my body. If my colon is not working optimally, then the rest of my body will not be working optimally either. The key to getting healthy is healing my colon and my gut and cleaning out my garbage.

Imagine I have a house and instead of taking my garbage to the curb every week, I put it inside my spare bedroom. Every week for years and years, I pile up my garbage inside my spare bedroom. Eventually this toxic room will stink up and toxify the rest of my house. Quickly there will be mold, bugs and critters that will start forming in this room. It won't matter how much air freshener I spray inside my house, my toxic garbage room will ruin my whole home environment.

It's the same with my body. Eventually my toxic stinky colon, will effect the rest of my system. So I clean out my system and begin feeling amazing!!!!

A LOVE NOTE FROM PETRA: "I have zero crap inside my body to cleanse anyway", is the funniest lie you will tell yourself. Having guided hundreds of cleansers, I know for a fact, WE ALL HAVE OLD CRAP INSIDE US, even the skinny people. We all have extra crap that is clogging up our system and slowly making us sick. So let's finally get rid of the old emotional and physical crap so we are thriving in health, energy and vitality again. My JUICY cleansers are always so shocked at how much fecal matter is coming out of them, when they haven't eaten solid food for days and weeks. This shows us that we have excess waste and toxic garbage stored in our colons and hiding in every bend of our intestines including the little pockets that have formed for storage. On one of my 10 day JUICY cleanses in Bali, I had a black hard poo about 5 inches long that came out of my body during my 2nd colonic. I had not eaten any food for 10 days and this old poo got flushed out of my system. The colon hydro therapist and I knew, it had been lodged somewhere in my system for a many years. Yipeee I got the toxic sludge out.

- - ♥ - -

CHAPTER 3

HISTORY OF CLEANSING / FASTING

S TOPPING THE INTAKE OF FOOD, also called fasting, has been practiced for centuries in the name of religion / culture and is still going on today. Almost every major religion encourages fasting which during certain momentous moments, people stop eating or drinking for a period of 24 or 48 hours to honor their Gods.

Unfortunately these religious fasting breaks are not health focused, so people break their fast with a huge glutinous and not so healthy feast. Since these fasts are for cultural and religious reasons, the healing possibilities of fasting do not get considered. There is a disconnect to fasting and what it can do for our body.

Ideally instead of just fasting for an external God presence, I could start fasting to honor the internal God presence that lives in each one of us. I can start honoring this Divine body temple that is taking such good care of me and giving my consciousness a place to live while we cruise around earth. As most religions are fasting for an outer source of power, I can fast for my inner source of power. I can stop eating or lighten my eating habits for myself, honoring the miracle that is ME. Then if I fast for religious reasons, I can create a whole body healing and spiritual God experience all in one.

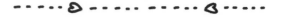

CHAPTER 4

CLEANSE LEVEL OPTIONS

LEVEL 1 ~ ~ Water only

LEVEL 2 ~ ~ Add Coconut Water

LEVEL 3 ~ ~ Add Juices & Lemon Water

LEVEL 4 ~ ~ Add Super Cleansers

LEVEL 5 ~ ~ Add Chlorophyll & Algaes

LEVEL 6 ~ ~ Add Teas, Mylks & Green Smoothies

LEVEL 7 ~ ~ Add Raw Soups

LEVEL 8 ~ ~ Add Fatty Smoothies

LEVEL 9 ~ ~ Add Salads

There are many ways I can cleanse depending on the results I want to achieve. I don't have to go on a JUICY food cleanse to cleanse. Stopping or reducing something I am eating that is not good for my body for a period of time is also a cleanse. If I stop eating meat and processed food for a few weeks, I am cleansing. I am cleansing my body from having to work hard to digest meat and processed crap for a few weeks. My body will be happier, healthier and have more energy. This level of cleansing will help my body, but in order to flush out my toxins and old garbage, I have to drink JUICY liquids.

I can also cleanse by stopping wheat, gluten and dairy for a few weeks. I can gently cleanse my body by stopping soda pop, GMO toxic potato chips, food colorings and synthetic ingredients. If I stop drinking alcohol and smoking cigarettes for a few weeks, my body will be cleansing. The type of cleansing I choose to do is up to me. I am brave and start SOME KIND of cleansing and do it as often as possible.

These cleanse options might feel advanced yet are simple to do. The water only cleanse is the most intense, yet the most basic to do. I drink just water. I read through this book and feel into which cleanse type feels right for me. Anything I choose to add or take away for my JUICY cleanse is up to me. I create my cleanse as it feels right for me. I have been given a guidance system so I have more power to do so.

During my cleanse, I am gentle with myself. Cleansing will most likely give me energy, yet it is still very important to rest. I might feel drained or I might feel energized, it will depend on the kind of cleanse I choose and the amount of cleansing my body needs. Everyone's experience is unique and each time I cleanse it will be a unique experience. The lower the Cleanse Level number I choose, the more rest I will need. For example, with a water cleanse I might want to sleep all day and give my body time to regenerate or I might need an hour nap but can go to work, do daily activities, exercise and socialize. As I cleanse, I will notice that my mind is sharper, my dreams more vivid and my memory stronger. As I release the toxins that are polluting my body, my organs will begin functioning better.

Giving my body a break from everything and feeding it a flood of nutrition, will allow my body's own self healing mechanism to kick into action. My body will naturally heal me of any dis-ease and bring me back to full alignment as it was designed to do. When I stop my intake of toxins and give the body a break, it will naturally start healing me back to my most optimal state.

I remember to cleanse the mental and emotional at the same time as I cleanse on the physical level. I am an energetic being that is storing old energy in my system, so letting this old energetic crap go is just as important as the physical crap I am releasing. Issues live in my tissues so as I cleanse, my body will begin to release and bring to the surface old stored up emotional baggage. I allow myself the time and space to release this. An emotional release will help me get skinnier, healthier and happier. When my mind, heart and soul are covered with emotional baggage, my body is denser. By releasing the emotional along with the physical, I will feel extremely lighter and freer. I will lose excess weight, my clothes will fit better and

I will feel happier looking in the mirror. On an emotional level, my life will feel more inspiring and worth living.

I do this cleanse for me so I feel good in my skin and love who is looking back at me in the mirror.

A LOVE NOTE FROM PETRA: Actually the most intense and most basic cleanse is a Dry Fast, where we wouldn't eat or drink anything and just breathe air. Yes people do it and it is safe, but I would not recommend it. I would prefer you infuse your body with JUICY liquids as humanity is actually massively dehydrated and at the stem of most sickness is dehydration. Hydrate and heal yourself at the same time. If you want to do a dry fast, then start with a juice cleanse, then transition to a water cleanse and then dry cleanse. This will be much easier for your body to transition. I believe in juices, smoothies, superfood cleansers, coconut water, herbal teas and spring water for cleansing. This is how I guide my JUICY retreats and online JUICY coaching programs. I think you will be surprised of how good you feel.

Start at Cleanse Level #9 if you have never cleansed before. You will feel very full, have an abundance of yummy food to drink and eat. Choose Cleanse Level #8 if you can release chewing food and drink liquids only. You will also feel full and nourished. Most JUICY cleanses & detox retreats I lead are Cleanse Level #6.

When I do my own personal cleansing, I usually start at Cleanse Level #9 and work my way down from there. The first few days I might eat salads and raw soups, then move my way to liquids only, then juices only, then coconut water only and then water only. I like to have fatty coconut or almond mylks in the evening to help me with my late night appetite. I also like to make fatty cashew or avocado raw soups during the first few days to help me with my hunger and then transition to no fibre juices.

How I move along the cleanse scale is up to me and it changes with every cleanse I do. It also changes depending on the effect I desire to achieve in my body.

- - ♡ - -

CLEANSE LEVEL 1 ~ ~ WATER ONLY

Drink water only. Ideally lead into a water cleanse by doing a JUICY cleanse first to make the transition easier. Or I just go for it, if this is the level of expedited healing I am after. On a water cleanse I become more sensitive to my environment and I might need a lot more rest. Sleep will be really essential in my healing and I might want to spend more time alone focusing energy on myself. This cleanse is safe and my body can survive without food. How much water I drink is up to me, yet ideally I space out my water drinking timing for every hour to keep me more satiated and on track. This cleanse level will kick my body into ketosis for expedited healing. Petra believes in giving the body lots of nutrition in the form of green juices and prefers healing the body with a green JUICY cleanse instead of jumping into a water cleanse. She suggests I transition into a water cleanse after drinking green juices for several days.

CLEANSE LEVEL 2 ~ ~ ADD COCONUT WATER

Also drink coconut water. Fresh coconuts are better than the carton / bottled versions which are usually pasteurized. If I am drinking bottled coconut water then I read the ingredients and buy only the pure brands. Some brands add sugar and others preservative chemicals. I buy carton instead of cans if I have choice, to avoid putting metals into my body. Coconut water will add more minerals and natural sugar into my system and ease up my hunger cravings than if I drank water only. On this cleanse I could still be very sensitive and not have much energy or I could be flying high energized and vibrant. My journey will be up to me. Coconut water is 99.9% the same as my human blood, so drinking lots of coconut water is like giving my self a blood transfusion.

CLEANSE LEVEL 3A ~ ~ ADD GREEN VEGGIE JUICES (NO FRUIT) + LEMON WATER + HERBAL TEAS

Also drink green veggie juices, lemon water and herbal teas. This cleanse is commonly used for cancer healing. Since there is no fruit or sugar in this cleanse, the body expedites its healing. Cancer loves sugar and gets bigger every time it eats some. This cleanse gives the cells tons of nutrition and helps release cancer cells out of my body. This cleanse is also great for candida, as it starves the yeast fungus out of my body which is also fed by sugar. Also drink green juice shooters of wheatgrass, barley grass, papaya leaf, hemp leaf, maringa leaf or other freshly juiced green grasses or leaves. They are a concentrated rich dose of chlorophyll and quickly alkaline and detoxify my body. They also quickly boost my immune system and are high in protein.

CLEANSE LEVEL 3B ~ ~ ADD ROOT VEGGIE JUICES + FRUIT VEGGIE JUICES

Also drink fruit and root vegetable juices. To expedite my healing process, I continue to limit the amount of sugar I drink. Most guided detoxes and juice cleansing programs, use this cleanse level. Make green juices adding in apples / pineapple / oranges / etc to add sweetness and make my green juices taste yummier. I don't make fruit only juices. Fruit juices with no fibre are high in sugar and spike up the sugar levels in my body. Drinking sugary juices is not ideal for cleansing, healing or a healthy lifestyle. It is healthier for me to blend in raw leafy greens into my fruity juices. My juices remain fruity in taste and I won't spike my glycemic levels as much. For example, I can make fresh orange juice and blend leafy greens into it to balance the sugar levels and increase my healing potential.

Some restaurants or juice bars add sugar to juices to increase the sweetness and make the juices taste better. In Bali this is a common practice in the local restaurants. I always request no additional sugars be added. Fruit juice examples are watermelon, orange, grapefruit, papaya and pineapple. Root vegetable examples are carrot and beet, which also convert to sugar inside my body.

A LOVE NOTE FROM PETRA: A special note about beet and carrot juice for cancer healing. There are many stories of people healing themselves from cancer, drinking just beet or just carrot juice, or a combination of the two. The nutrition inside these two vegetables is powerful enough to heal cancer even if these root vegetables convert to sugar in the body. My recommendation for cancer healing is to also add chlorophyll from green raw food to expedite and support healing. Chlorophyll is 99.9% the same as our blood (hemoglobin). So drinking lots of green liquid will naturally clean our blood and rebuild our system.

- - ♥ - -

CLEANSE LEVEL 4 ~ ~ ADD IN SUPER CLEANSERS

Also drink super food cleansers to take the toxins out of the body faster. Super food cleanser examples are diatomaceous earth, activated charcoal, bentonyte clay, psyllium husk, hydrogen peroxide and baking soda. These super food cleansers bind to the toxins in my body and scrape them out. They also help alkaline my body. If I want a simple cleanse, then I don't add them in. If I want a deeper cleanse, then I eat these super food cleansers with care and understanding of how to truly use them. They are powerful and can really support my cleansing regime and also my new JUICY lifestyle.

CLEANSE LEVEL 5 ~ ~ ADD CHLOROPHYLL AND ALGAES

Also now drink more chlorophyll (in the semi processed form). Chlorophyll coming from sea weed algaes like spirulina, chlorella, liquid chlorophyll and blue / green algae called blue magick. These super seaweeds come from the oceans and lakes and are packed full of nutrition. Some smell a little like dirty socks but they ARE GOOD FOR ME! Heehehee! I can try them in the powder form to create them into lemony drinks. I mix a teaspoon of green powder with spring water and lemon juice in a glass jar and shake it up. I will be surprised that my lemony chlorophyll drink tastes really good. The lemon hides the flavor of the greens and the drink taste very refreshing.

Having green powders on hand is great when I don't have access to green juices or green smoothies in my every day healthy lifestyle. They are also great for traveling, road trips, having in my desk at work and in my gym work out bag. All I need is water, lemon juice and green powder to make myself an amazing easy healthy green drink. I can usually get lemon wedges in most restaurants and bars to support me while I travel.

A LOVE NOTE FROM PETRA: I don't add these green powders to smoothies or juices as some people do, because it makes my whole drink taste less appealing. I would prefer to have a yummy smoothie or juice and then have a separate lemony green chlorophyll drink.

- - ♥ - -

CLEANSE LEVEL 6 ~ ~ ADD TEA ELIXIRS, NUT MYLKS AND GREEN SMOOTHIES

Also drink tea elixirs, nut mylks and green smoothies. At this level, I can eat fatty drinks and fiber rich smoothies to satiate my hunger and make my cleanse much easier. Petra starts her cleansers at this level when they want a gentler and easier JUICY cleanse. If I have cancer, candida or diabetes, then I will want to make savory green smoothies instead of fruity ones to avoid the sugar.

Drinking fiber does take some of my digesting power but because it is blended in a smoothie, the work my body has to do is minimal. I drink the fiber green smoothies to scrape out my intestines like a scrub brush. The fiber also helps me grow good bacteria in my gut and helps me have a more balanced body system.

CLEANSE LEVEL 7 ~ ~ ADD RAW SOUPS

Add in hot or cold raw food soups. A raw soup is not cooked, all veggies and green leafy greens are raw and blended in a blender with hot or cold water. Use hot water, cold water, coconut mylk or cashew milk as a base. By blending all the ingredients, I am still liquid cleansing and giving my body a break from digesting. Since the fiber is blended and broken down, the body has much less to digest.

Raw soup ingredients are a combination of raw veggies, leafy greens, avocados, cashews, nut mylks, miso paste, chili paste, oils and spices. They are a great way to BEGIN CLEANSING and are also really quick meals for my upcoming JUICY lifestyle. I can use hot water and my raw vegetables remain raw but are now just heated. Hot raw soups are an easy way to make quick meals, start cleanses, maintain nutrition levels and eat life force. Most restaurant soups are over boiled and the vegetable nutrition is cooked out. When I use hot water, raw vegetables and a blender, I create a hot soup that is nutrition packed and full of colon scraping fiber.

I can also use a cooked soup as my base and up level it. For example, I put cooked pumpkin soup into a blender, add in raw spinach and blend it up. I now have a pumpkin soup that is full of green nutrition. The more greens the better of course.

A LOVE NOTE FROM PETRA: I usually start my personal juice cleanses at this level. I drink juices throughout the day and add hot raw soups for the first few days to make my cleansing gentler. By day 3, I release the soups and move into Cleanse Level #6 and make my way down the Levels as I feel.

- - ♥ - -

CLEANSE LEVEL 8 ~ ~ ADD FAT PROTEIN SMOOTHIES

Add smoothies made with protein powders, coconut oil, coconut meat, avocado, almond butter, cacao butter, coconut milk or coconut yogurt. This Cleanse Level is THE BEST if I am new to cleansing but want to do liquids only. I have been brainwashed to believe that fat is bad for me and I should eat everything low fat. This is a lie, fat is good for me as long as it is the healthy kind. My brain is made of fat and so are my organs. Good fat can also help take the bad fat out of my body. Eating a teaspoon daily of good quality coconut oil CAN MAKE ME SKINNY and heal my gut! This cleanse level is the easiest way to ease into liquid cleansing.

- - ♡ - -

CLEANSE LEVEL 9 ~ ~ ADD KICK ASS BIG BOWL SALADS

Add in eating HEALTHY salads. At this level I drink liquids and eat kick ass big bowl salads to fill me up and CLEANSE ME VERY GENTLY. If I am very new to cleansing or eating healthy, then this is the BEST PLACE TO START. I can eat and drink healthy for 7 days. Although my body is using some of it's energy for digesting the salads, it is still only digesting raw vegetables which will process quickly and give me lots of vitamins, life force energy and fiber to scrape me out. My body will love me.

A kick ass big bowl salad is any combination of various green leaves, chopped veggies, nuts, seeds and a healthy amazing dressing. I make my salad fresh or if I buy a salad, I ask about the ingredients of the salad dressing. Usually a salad is super healthy and the dressing is a toxic mix of crappy vegetable oils, sugar, high fructose corn syrup and preservatives. If I have no healthy dressing options, I ask for lemon, olive oil and salt. Raw apple cider vinegar and olive oil is a great salad dressing also. The apple cider vinegar needs to be raw, unpasteurized and have the "mother" bits floating in it. Most favorite brand is Braggs. Apple cider vinegar is very alkaline for my body and very healthy. Other vinegars like white or balsamic are acidic for my body and not as healthy. I use lemons, limes or apple cider vinegar for my dressings and also add them to water to make alkaline morning drinks. Alkaline drinks and kick ass big bowl salads are essential diet staples to living my upcoming JUICY lifestyle.

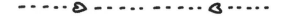

CHAPTER 5

THIS TOO IS
A CLEANSE

ANYTIME I CUT OUT SOMETHING THAT IS NOT beneficial for my body it is considered cleansing too. If it is harmful, hard to digest or creates an allergic reaction inside my body, then it will serve me to remove it for a period of time or for the rest of my life. Wink! Wink! The standard American diet or the outdated food pyramid, I have been brainwashed to believe, is actually quite harmful for my body. When I cut out gluten, meat, dairy and sugar out of my diet for a period of time, quickly I will feel amazing. Most likely I will have more energy, my allergies will clear up, my nose stops being stuffy every morning, my bowels work better, my joints hurt less and I feel a younger version of myself.

I go for it!!!! I try removing some of these foods out of my lifestyle to feel the effects in my body. I can also slowly introduce them back in after my cleanse and see how they make me feel. This can be an interesting experiment, remove certain food and introduce it back in to gauge my body's response.

Meat, gluten, white sugar, processed sugar, dairy, white flour, soy, canola oil, stress, alcohol, cigarettes, processed food and preservatives do not have a place in my JUICY lifestyle. They are natural allergens to my body and my body sees them as invaders. My white blood cells actually begin attacking these invaders and my body has to work extra hard to protect me. When I cut these foods out, I will notice an improvement in my energy, my digestive power and my joint health. The way these foods are created now compared to the old days, has created them to be very toxic for my body. There are many alternative sources of these types of foods that are much healthier for my body and I am inspired to try them. If I choose to get a proper food allergy test, I will most likely find that my body is actually allergic to gluten, dairy, eggs and soy.

MORE GREAT CLEANSE OPTIONS FOR ME TO TRY:

For 7 or 14 or 21 days....
- Cut out gluten
- Cut out processed sugar
- Cut out dairy
- Cut out processed lab food and eat only whole earth food
- Cut out meat
- Cut out alcohol
- Cut out stress and self hate
- Eat as much liquid food as possible
- Eat lots of raw food with very little cooked food
- In the mirror tell myself -"I love you"

CHAPTER 6

HOW MANY DAYS DO I CLEANSE?

CAN CLEANSE FOR 3 + DAYS AS a GREAT START. Ideally 7 + days is the best as it usually takes the first 3 days for my body to get used to cleansing and to start feeling really good. For most people, the first 3 days may be an emotional battle of not eating or the fearful feelings of hunger. By day 4, most people notice that they feel great, are not hungry and realize cleansing is easier than they thought.

It is also good to do a mini cleanses more frequently, like 1 day every week for several months. Perhaps every Monday I just eat liquids and give my digestive system a break. Perhaps the first 3 days of the month I eat only raw food and liquids. Ideally I cleanse for 7 days once or twice per year. How often I cleanse is up to me based on the healing I desire.

The state of my health is up to me. I am receiving tools in this book to reverse all sickness and heal my body. How often I use these tools is up to me. If am sick or know I need some deep cleansing then I do a JUICY liquid cleanse for 14 days or for 1 month. The more green juices and water I drink, the more my body will heal. I use my internal guidance system, to know what is right for me.

I remember that removing wheat, gluten, dairy, meat, alcohol, cigarettes and stress out of my life for a few weeks or few months is also a wonderful way to cleanse my body. So I move towards a new JUICY lifestyle that I can make work and that I am willing to commit to.

Eating smaller portions than before is also a cleanse. Instead of stuffing my face with 1 big meal per day, it is better for me to eat a few smaller meals throughout the day. I stop eating when I am full instead of forcing myself to eat every bite. When I eat past my full limit, my stomach can't handle the amount of food and pushes the undigested food into my intestines to putrefy and rot.

Replacing my breakfast with a big green smoothie and replacing my lunch with a kick ass big bowl salad is a great cleanse too. In order for a green smoothie and kick ass salad cleanse to be effective, I have to do it consistently for a few weeks gradually making it a forever part of my new JUICY lifestyle.

CHAPTER 7

HOW WILL I FEEL?

N THE BEGINNING, I MIGHT HAVE THE LINGERING feeling of hunger. Yes, I might be physically hungry but if I drink enough liquids, my hunger pangs will only be emotional. It's not easy to say which comes first, either my belly signaling my mind that I am hungry or my mind telling my belly that it should be hungry because I have not eaten for hours.

Sometimes it is hard to let go of my preconditioned idea that I should be eating. Our bodies have been conditioned that if we are not eating, then something must be wrong. Maybe it comes from our ancestral times, when if we went long periods without food, we would die. So on some subconscious level, I fear that if I don't eat for 7 days, I might die. It is RIDICULOUS!!!

I am drinking nutrient dense and vitamin packed liquids that will fill me up and feed my body with everything I need. Giving up food is more of a mental game then it is a physical one. Sometimes when I am told that I can't have something, I want it even more. So I feed my body liquid every hour and reprogram my mind that I am safe and I am ok.

Overall during my JUICY cleanse, I should be feeling very good. If I drink often enough, I will feel full, have energy and be quite surprised how easy cleansing is.

It is also possible that in the first few days of my cleanse, I feel nauseous or unsettled in my belly. When the toxins start releasing out of my system, I might feel a little off. Also if my body is very acidic, then alkaline chlorophyll rich green drinks can make me want to throw up. I say YIPEEE if my body throws up. It is not the green juice my body is throwing up, but the toxins that the green juice stirred up. So it is better that the crap be out of my body, then inside poisoning me.

It is also possible that in the latter part of my cleansing week, I feel dizzy when I stand up as my blood sugar levels have dropped. Again I am safe. If I am concerned, I can add in more fruity juices during my JUICY cleanse. My blood sugar levels will regulate on this cleanse as my body reboots itself to a new healthier system.

I might get headaches or feel flu like symptoms during the first few days of my cleanse. Toxins are being released from my cells and start swimming around in my system. My body loves me so it has hidden the toxins inside my cells to keep them away from the rest of my body system. When my body knows I am cleansing, it releases all the stored up toxins into my blood stream and lymphatic fluid, so I can start flushing them out. I might also have stinky breath, stinky body odor or a very mucous covered tongue as my toxins are getting out of my system.

I do not stop my cleanse just because I feel these little discomforts in my body. There is more discomfort in me getting sick if I do not cleanse my body. Of course I listen to my intuition and act on what feels right for me. And I know that the nauseous or headachy feelings will go away within a day or two, as I get rid of the toxic crap in my body that is actually making me sick.

Some people think they have to stop the green juices or green smoothies because they feel a headache or a flu coming on. It is not the green juice that is making me sick, it is the toxins that are inside my body that the green juice is cleaning out. The toxins are making me feel sick, not the green juice. If left alone, these toxins will stay tucked away inside my cells slowly causing my body damage. I might not notice them at first but eventually they will cause me aches, pains, rashes and diseases. Eventually they will build up and cause me bigger and bigger sickness. So I cleanse and flush the toxins out of my body now.

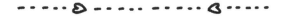

I GET RID OF TOXIC CRAP
THAT IS MAKING MY BODY SICK

I GIVE MY BODY
THIS TIME TO HEAL

I AM WORTH IT

- - ♡ - -

CHAPTER 8

RESTING & SLEEPING

THIS JUICY FOOD CLEANSE IS AN OPPORTUNITY to connect to my body. I am gentle, kind and loving to my body that is working hard to heal me in every moment and working especially hard during this cleansing process.

I may feel tired during the first few days of my JUICY cleanse or I might feel tired on the back end of my week. One of the most important things to do during this cleanse is give myself permission to rest and to sleep.

I will attempt going to sleep early and getting at least 8 hours of sleep during this JUICY cleanse to super heal. My body really focuses on my healing while I sleep. If I am a late owl and usually burn the candle at both ends, then I try sleeping more during this cleanse to speed up my healing process.

While I sleep, my body is pushing all my toxins to the bowel and tongue areas for morning clean up. While I sleep, my body is in restoration mode. Sleeping gives my body time to do the necessary clean up. When I eat food too late, my body spends all night digesting rather than cleaning and healing. When I eat late, I wake up feeling tired as my body had been working all night instead of resting.

Power naps can rock my world during this JUICY cleanse and also during my new JUICY lifestyle, so I try them. I set my phone alarm for 22 or 44 minutes and lay down, for a much needed reboot and rejuvenation. I might not fall asleep, that's ok, I am giving my body time to rest and relax.

I promise to add more restful rejuvenating sleep into my life starting now...

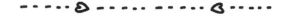

CHAPTER 9

MEDITATING

NOW LET'S MEDITATE! If meditation has not been a regular part of my life then – I TRY IT! Meditation is a quiet moment of time for myself and a time to remember that I am a powerful human walking around on planet earth. If I don't know how to meditate, then this chapter will give me some guidance. Yet ultimately meditation is closing my eyes and connecting to my inner self and to my inner world. I get quiet and listen to what my mind, body, heart and soul are saying to me. I get quiet to listen for downloads of information and ideas from the universe. I get quiet and internally spend time empowering myself with healthy self talk.

I can Google "guided meditations" on Youtube, close my eyes and listen. Sometimes having someone talk me through meditations and visualizations is easier than just sitting there trying to keep my mind empty. Being guided is great a technique that can help me drop in to myself faster and deeper.

The most important part of meditation, no matter what style I choose, is close my eyes, be still and take this time for myself. I am worth it!

I may think that I have to quiet the monkey mind while I meditate and this can be the most difficult part. It is not about quieting this constant dialogue within, but slowing it down enough to witness it. I close my eyes and allow myself the time to see what I am constantly saying inside my own head. Are my thoughts positive or negative? What constant belief am I having? What keeps spinning on the inside that needs to be released or transformed? I use my meditation as a time to slow the voice down and be a witness to myself.

Setting an alarm on my phone or listening to a guided meditation can be helpful to create a timed container for me to sit in. Instead of needing to check the time, I can wait for the buzzer and relax into the moment.

- - ♥ - -

SOME WAYS I MAY MEDITATE. I CLOSE MY EYES AND ...

1. Listen to guided meditations.
2. Say empowering statements to myself to reprogram my inner belief system.
3. Visualize a healing conversation with someone I wish to forgive.
4. Dream up my perfect incredible life 3 years from now in full detail.
5. Imagine my most amazing day from morning till I go to bed in full detail.
6. Breathe in and out, filling every crevasse of my body skin bag with air.
7. Sit and witness what thoughts or conversations are being played in my head.
8. Visualize a dream I wish to manifest. I feel it. I am in it. I see it as already so.
9. Connect to my body. I breathe deep and expand my chest. What is my body saying?
10. Connect to my inner child. I feel the little 7 year old inside of me. What does it need?
11. Put on some music. Move my body. I am flexible. I move. I breathe. I keep my eyes closed.

I remember to be gentle with myself, love myself and give myself the space that is needed for healing. I am cleansing on a physical, mental and emotional level so I remember how miraculous my body is and I thank it for healing me today.

My AMAZING MIRACULOUS body is working for my greatest healing and vitality in every moment, doing this JUICY cleanse is ME supporting MY body with the healing it is already attempting to accomplish daily. I give my body a break from digesting. I release the stress, anger, resentment and wounding that might still be living in my body. I rest, relax and let go of as much stress as possible. I connect to my heart and to my inner intuition, that is speaking to me in all moments. I listen and take action to fulfill my inner deepest desires.

MY BODY LOVES ME
MY BODY IS A MIRACULOUS HEALING MACHINE
I AM MADE UP OF ENERGY
I AM LOVED
I AM SAFE
I AM HEALTHY
I AM WHOLE
I AM ENOUGH
I AM WORTHY
I AM LOVE

- - ♡ - -

CHAPTER 10

EXERCISE & STRETCHING

URING THIS JUICY CLEANSE I MIGHT FEEL super energized and go daily to the gym, yoga studio or go running, or I might not want to do any physical activity as my body wants more rest time. How I feel is very individual to me so I listen to my body and go for the ride.

Most likely I will have energy throughout my cleanse. I rest, have power naps and do lighter exercise. It feels good for my body to move and it feels equally good to give my body time to rest. I am always gentle with myself and I choose what feels right for me in every moment. Only I know and only I can choose what works for me.

I incorporate light exercise and stretching daily to move

everything inside my body. I can find Youtube videos on yin yoga, restorative yoga or mat stretching, if I need a teacher to follow. Or I can also put on some yummy music, close my eyes and move around on the carpet or my yoga mat as my body naturally wants to move. I listen to my intuition, surrender and move. I might think I need to be guided but my body knows how it wants to move. Now it is time for me to listen.

I ADD stretching to my new JUICY lifestyle and do it daily for the rest of my life! Most likely I am sitting or standing somewhere all day and my body is tight. The more I can stretch my muscles and lengthen my body, the more my body energy can flow. So I don't worry if I don't know how to do yoga or how to do certain exercises, I just stretch my muscles and expand my body. I stretch my body and breathe in lots of oxygen into these new expanded areas. The more oxygen I take into my body, the more healing will take place. So I expand, I breathe and my body LOVEs me!

Daily I get on the floor, on my carpet or my yoga mat and stretch. I am old when I am rigid, tight and inflexible. I create flexibility and agility in my body, I create YOUTHENING. I add in DAILY stretching into my thoughts and make it a part of my DAILY life. I promise this to myself. I love myself and I love my body.

THE 5 MOST IMPORTANT AREAS I WILL STRETCH ARE:

1. HIPS – most likely I hold all my emotion and blocked energy in my hip and groin area. So I stretch this. I self massage and push into these areas to loosen up the tight pain. I release blocked energy here. If I have a partner, I ask them to help me stretch or massage this area. I invest in massages for myself. I am worth it.

2. SPINE – the key to longevity is a healthy spine. When my spine is flexible, I am youthful. So I bend, I stretch and I twist my spine every day to create more mobility in this area.

3. ANKLES AND WRISTS – these areas work a lot for me throughout the day. So I rotate them. I move them in circles. They might crack so I keep rotating them to get the tightness out.

4. NECK – this area holds up my fabulous smart head and can hold a lot of tension. So I turn my head, I stretch my neck and I self massage this area as often as possible. I alternate carrying my bag on different shoulders. I straighten up my spine when I walk and sit. I notice the posture I hold when I type on my computer, play with my cell phone and watch TV. Am I hunching over? I pull my head back and create more fluidity in my neck.

5. CHEST – open this area up. Maybe I am hunched over. Sometimes out of laziness for a proper posture but a lot of the time because I am unconsciously protecting my heart. When I straighten up and stretch my heart out, it can feel

vulnerable and not safe. I push my chest out anyway, open up my arms and push my heart out. I open this delicate area of my body and I am safe. A door frame is a great exercise machine to stretch my arms and chest as it is the perfect size.

Here are some fun visual examples of stretches if I need further guidance. Ideally I close my eyes and listen to what my body wants to do. It will direct me on how it wants to stretch and move. I LISTEN!!!

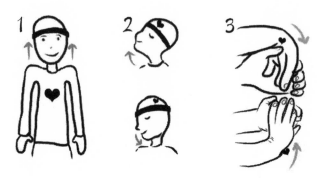

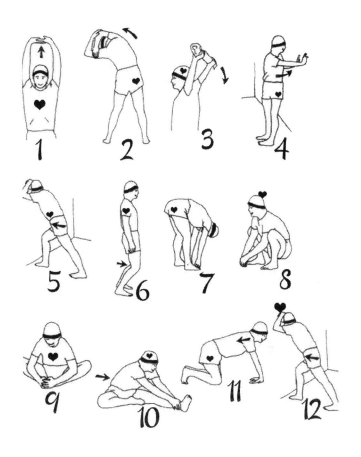

I ADD STRETCHING TO MY
NEW JUICY LIFESTYLE AND
DO IT DAILY
FOR THE REST OF MY LIFE!

- - ♡ - -

CHAPTER 11

FOOD IS A JOURNEY

MOST OF US HAVE EMOTIONAL ATTACHMENTS to food. We are attached to how it can make us feel and what we think food can do for us emotionally. The thought of giving up this energy may feel very scary for me. Maybe food is my safety, my comfort, my sense of love and also maybe my greatest punisher. I can use food to either love myself or I can use it to punish myself.

Food helps me to stuff down my emotions when I don't want to feel them. A big pasta meal is going to help me stuff down my emotions easier than a salad. It's going to make me feel safe, comfortable and give me that full belly feeling that maybe I associate with security.

Unknowingly, most mothers lock their children into emotional food dependency bonds. They show their children to avoid feeling their emotions using food as a way of feeling safe. If something doesn't work out or a child is sad, then mom makes her child's favorite dish or bakes sugary goodies to comfort her baby and put a smile on their face.

I am ready for more emotional healing so I allow my JUICY cleanse to bring up the emotions, hurts, regrets, resentments and anger that I might have living inside of me. Feelings, hurts, anger, resentment, pain, regrets, shame, guilt and desires that I have been stuffing down for years, not wanting to feel before. I use this JUICY cleanse to let go of the crap that is no longer serving me but still living in my body and causing me harm. I might not currently feel it or realize it is in there, yet if I haven't released it, healed it or forgiven it, it is in there. Slowly behind the scenes, underneath my every day life, these feelings are robbing me of my energy. These pains, resentments and angers are slowly poisoning me and energetically making me feel unbalanced.

During this cleanse, I let it all come up. I am brave and I allow myself to FEEL IT!!!! As I feel it then I can heal it. Breathe, cry, beat a pillow, go lock myself in my car and scream. Release the old stuff so I can be lighter, healthier and happier.

Anger, resentment, hate and lack of forgiveness create sickness and premature aging in my body. Feeling negative energy towards someone is like drinking poison and expecting the other to die. Slowly I poison myself every day and lower my quality of life. I am in control and in charge of my internal emotional state. Only I can release, forgive and heal. Only I can choose to stop my internal suffering and bring more peace into my life. I use this JUICY cleanse time to get in touch with my emotions and my feelings that are no longer serving me AND I GET RID OF THEM!

I take time to experience my emotions during this cleanse and continue to experience them for the rest of my life. I am a whole being made up of energy. If the energy I am holding in my body is negative and low vibration, then this will affect all parts of my body and my life. I remember my wholeness and choose to release the old stagnation. It might be scary or feel painful at first to face the dark that is within me yet I will feel so much better once I have healed it and will wonder why I hung on to it for so long.

Can I remember a time where I felt so nauseous in my stomach that I wanted to throw up? That feeling of nausea and illness felt so terrible, yet when I finally threw up and released the energy, I felt so much better, lighter and freer. This is the same with my emotional cleansing state. To experience these emotions will feel uncomfortable and scary, but once I allow them to be healed and released out of my body, I will feel amazing.

So JUICY cleansing is a journey into my emotions. It is an opportunity to feel them and heal them.

JUICY food and raw food are the fastest ways to my evolution and consciousness expansion. If I am on a spiritual journey and desire to AWAKEN and EXPAND faster, then I cleanse my body to remove the toxic build up and add more JUICY raw food to my lifestyle to continue the healing process.

Juices and raw food are light and when eaten lighten up my body. Cooked food is heavy and when eaten weighs down my body and the energy inside my body.

I can understand and imagine that right? I eat a salad or drink a juice, I feel light and energized. I eat a big pasta meal or a big pizza, I feel heavy and tired.

So if I want to feel lighter, happier, brighter and more energized then I start this JUICY cleanse right now and then continue this healthier eating into my new JUICY lifestyle. If I want energy, I need to eat energy. Juices and raw food are full of the sun's energy. This energy gets transferred into my body and makes me feel energized.

The plant leaves collect the sun's energy and give this energy to all the fruits and veggies of the plant. When I drink and eat raw fruits and vegetables, I am directly eating sunshine energy. When I drink and eat raw fruits and vegetables, I am also eating life force energy. The plant is still growing, fruits are ripening, veggies are getting bigger, they are alive and eating this life force energy makes me feel energized.

The juices, smoothies and raw meals also use less digesting power and are full of life force, so they vibrate energetically much faster and higher. The more juices I drink, the more raw food I eat, the more I will vibrate at a higher frequency. My body mass energy will no longer be as dense and heavy and I will be lighter and more levitated. The more light my body is, the more light my body will emit. I will glow and people will wonder, "what are you doing? I want some of that!"

So I HEAL MY EMOTIONS! I lighten up! I shine the light that I am, inside my skin bag. I am brave and I can do this!

MORE HELP TO HEAL MY EMOTIONS...

1. Allow them to be. Feel them in my body and my heart. Feel safe knowing I am ok. Allow myself to fully feel and maybe relive some of these past experiences.

2. Recognize I am ok. This was the past. Knowing I am safe right here, right now.

3. Forgive. Let go. Consciously choose to release. Even if I don't know how, I ask the universe or God to take it from me.

Petra's first book *I AM AMAZING – A No Nonsense Self Love Guide To Remember Your Greatness And Rock Out Your Life* will be of great help. It is full of exercises and mind expansions to support my inner healing, forgiving and letting go. I can buy the book on Amazon.

Life is a journey and it keeps getting better and better every day. Life loves me and is always unfolding for my greatest expression of myself on this planet. Once I fully trust that the universe has my back and I fully love myself, then my experience of life will be better. Whether this is a good world or a bad world is up to me. I determine how I view myself and my outside experiences. The more I look for the good, the more I will find it. I drop into the gratitude of my life and all the good I have around me and the good within me. The more grateful I am, the more life will keep giving me more to be grateful for.

I am blessed and divinely taken care of. I am a conscious creator on this planet. I am the Queen / King of this life reality and how my life unfolds is up to me. Maybe I haven't been dealt the best cards to begin with or I may have experienced some tragic hurtful things, yet how I choose to live my life from this moment forward is now up to me. The quality of my health and my life is up to me. There is no one to blame any more. I am in charge. No one can determine my self worth or the inner state of my happiness. I trust in my journey and I trust in myself. I open up, let go of the crap and receive the goodness that is all around me. I am worthy and I deserve to be blissed out happy.

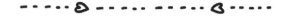

CHAPTER 12

HOW MUCH DO I LOVE MYSELF?

SELF LOVE – AHHHHH, THE MOST IMPORTANT healing and cleansing practice of them all.

I can drink green juices, eat supplements and do enemas until I am blue in the face BUT if I don't LOVE and adore myself, then I can't fully heal.

I can't be drinking green juices, saying hateful cruel things to myself and consider myself healthy. The fastest way to a happier life is to cleanse my MIND! Doing a JUICY cleanse is a great physical activity that holds the container for me to let go of the crap that I hold in my mind. All the limiting, self loathing, weak, victim consciousness, fearful, undeserving, hateful and cruel thoughts I think inside my head towards myself and others HAVE GOT TO GO!!!

My greatest journey on this planet is to my TRUE SELF LOVE state!   At the end of my time, I believe I will ask myself, "did I love myself enough that I allowed myself to fully open up and have the greatest, fullest, most abundant life possible?   Did I allow myself to fully receive with an open heart all the riches of the world or did I keep feeding myself the belief that I was unworthy and not ENOUGH, so I withheld from myself the ability to fully manifest all I deserve in my life?   How silly of me!"

This is my BIG WORK and MOST REWARDING WORK.   RADICAL SELF LOVE and becoming my OWN best friend!!!

Connecting to myself and to my soul is my LIFE'S GREATEST JOURNEY.   I start adoring myself today, more than I ever have before!

Here is a COOL tool that will help me expedite my SELF LOVE journey.   I will master it and do it for the rest of my life.

GRAB A MIRROR AND START LOOKING AT MYSELF ...

It might feel silly at first, I might hate it, I might hate who is looking back at me, I might not want to do it or think I am crazy for trying.

I DO IT ANYWAY!!!

1. Watch the thoughts that come up as I look at myself in the mirror.

2. Notice the things I say to myself. Notice the critical judging, perhaps even cruel voice.

3. Now talk to myself out loud. Say hi to myself. Connect to myself. See myself. Praise myself. Love myself.

4. Appreciate myself.

5. Listen and witness myself.

No matter my age, it's time to start self love. It is a practice. So I keep practicing. I keep practicing. I keep practicing. I keep practicing. I keep loving myself. I am worth it.

I start saying hi to myself every morning when I see myself in the mirror. Wave, wink, smile, acknowledge my aliveness and be grateful the universe has breathed me another day. Connect to myself as I am my own best friend and best companion.

Become a witness to the words I speak to myself and about myself inside my head. I slow this internal conversation down enough so I can witness it, question it and then switch my self love belief system.

I commit to loving myself more and more every day. I commit to doing mirror work during my JUICY cleanse and for the rest of my life. I commit to taking care of myself and spending energy on my own self care. If I give and give to others, I then deplete myself. I deserve energy and care too. So I give to myself so I am filled up. Then from a full radiant place I can give to others. I love myself enough to give to myself first. I am the most important person in my life. I honor myself and remember my worth.

I SAY TO MYSELF OVER AND OVER AGAIN...

I LOVE MYSELF.
I AM PROUD OF MYSELF.
I ADORE MYSELF. I AM SO GRATEFUL TO BE ME.
I TAKE CARE OF MYSELF.
I FEED MYSELF THE BEST MOST NOURISHING
FOOD AND LIQUIDS.
I PUT MYSELF INTO THE KINDEST
MOST LOVING SITUATIONS.
I SURROUND MYSELF WITH THE MOST
AMAZING LOVING PEOPLE.
I TAKE AWESOME CARE OF MYSELF. I LOVE MYSELF.
I NURTURE MYSELF. I AM GRATEFUL TO BE ME.
I DON'T WANT TO BE ANYONE ELSE. I LOVE ME.
I AM PROUD OF ME. I AM BRAVE.
I HAVE COURAGE. I HAVE DETERMINATION
I AM CHOOSING BETTER.
I AM CHOOSING A HAPPIER HEALTHIER LIFE
I AM A SUPER STAR!

This incredible poem is by the FABULOUS Marianne Williamson from her book *A Return To Love*. Check out this JUICY woman's work! To make the poem more personal, the YOU has been changed to I.

I remember my LIGHT with every word I read.

MY DEEPEST FEAR...

My deepest fear is not that I am inadequate
My deepest fear is that I am powerful beyond measure
It is my light, not my darkness
That most frightens me
I ask myself
Who am I to be brilliant, gorgeous, talented, fabulous?
Actually, who am I not to be?
I am a child of God
My playing small does not serve the world
There's nothing enlightened about shrinking
So that other people won't feel insecure around me
I am meant to shine, as all children do.
I was born to make manifest the glory of God that is within me
It's not just in some of us; It's in everyone.
And as I let my own light shine,
I unconsciously give other people permission to do the same
As I am liberated from my own fear,
My presence automatically liberates others

This poem is by the BEAUTIFUL Rev. Safire Rose. It's a perfect reminder that letting go of my crap is my internal choice and only I choose when I do it. I am in charge of my life and I am powerful to let my crap go. I don't need permission from anyone. To personalize it, SHE has been changed to I.

I LET GO with every word I read.

I LET GO...

I let go. Without a thought or a word, I let go
I let go of the fear
I let go of the judgments
I let go of the confluence of opinions swarming around my head
I let go of the committee of indecision within me
I let go of all the 'right' reasons
Wholly and completely, without hesitation or worry
I just let go
I don't ask anyone for advice
I don't read a book on how to let go
I don't search the scriptures
I just let go
I let go of all of the memories that held me back
I let go of all of the anxiety that keeps me from moving forward
I let go of the planning and all of the calculations about
how to do it just right
I don't promise to let go
I don't journal about it

I don't write the projected date in my day timer
I make no public announcement and put no ad in the paper
I don't check the weather report or read my daily horoscope
I just let go
I don't analyze whether I should let go
I don't call my friends to discuss the matter
I don't utter one word
I just let go
No one is around when it happens
There is no applause or congratulations
No one is thanking or praising me
No one notices a thing
Like a leaf falling from a tree
I just let go
There is no effort
There is no struggle
It isn't good and it isn't bad
It is what it is and it is just that
In the space of letting go
I let it all be
A small smile comes over my face
A light breeze blows through me
And the sun and the moon shines forevermore...

I AM GRATEFUL TO BE ON THIS LIFE
JOURNEY WITH MYSELF....

I LOVE ME!

- - ♡ - -

CHAPTER 13

I AM POWERFUL

AM MORE POWERFUL THAN I HAVE BEEN LEAD to believe. My body's ability to self heal is more powerful than I have been lead to believe. My mind is the most powerful friend or foe that I have and it can be used for my greatest thriving or my greatest destruction on this planet.

My body is a self healing machine that is healing me in every moment. Without me having to do anything, my fingernails are growing, my hair is growing and my stomach is digesting my food. If I am a woman, I can grow a baby inside my body without me having to really do anything. I just trust and leave the miracle to nature. My body is miraculous and I am a miracle made of cosmic star dust walking around this magnificent planet. I have the gift of life and the universe is constantly breathing me.

Dropping into my magnificence and counting gratitude for my life, will be my fastest routes to healing, cleansing and living an extraordinary life. The more grateful I am for my existence on this planet, the more I will love my body and the more I will love myself. The more I love myself, the better I will take care of myself. It is time for me to take my life and my health into my hands. It is time for me to know that the quality of my life and my health is 100% my responsibility. No more victim consciousness. No more looking out there for someone or something to heal me or make me whole. I am whole. I am perfect and beautiful in this very moment. If I don't like something about myself or my life, then I fix it or change it. I am powerful. I can do or be anything I desire.

The thoughts I think, the words I say and the things I believe, shape my reality. Where ever I am right now in my life, is because I took myself there. I own it. I own my health. I own my mindfulness. I own my life.

STARTING RIGHT NOW!

I start this 7 + day JUICY food cleanse and take back the health of my body right now! My body is crying out and waiting for my help. I get on board the healthy train with my body and help myself feel absolutely amazing. I deserve it. I am worth it. My life is worth it. It is my birthright to be thriving on this planet in perfect health, total abundance and pure joyful bliss.

I say YES to this journey of my life and my health and I GO FOR IT! It's easy. I got my back. I can do this!

CHAPTER 14

SET MY INTENTION

SET AN INTENTION FOR MY JUICY CLEANSE NOW. An intention is a committed focus or desirable outcome for my cleanse. Perhaps I want to feel a certain way, have my body look a certain way, let go of a part of my life that no longer serves me or change an undesirable habit. What do I want to create through my JUICY cleanse? What relationships, illnesses or thought patterns do I desire to heal? How will I know if my JUICY cleanse is a success? I ask myself all these questions and more.

I get a journal and write down answers to these questions and to the questions being asked below. During my cleansing week, I will use my journal to write about the experiences and feelings I am having. I write down my life visions, lists of things I am grateful for and my big dreams. I write down my ideal life, describe my perfect partner and my perfect career. I write down in detail. I write it like it has already happened, like I already have it. I feel it in my body and believe it to be real.

I might have thought that this JUICY cleansing is only a physical act and it can be that for me. I can just drink juices, cleanse my body on the physical level and be very successful. Yet if I can add in the emotional and spiritual to my cleanse and to my life, I will see how much faster my life and my health improve. Issues live in my tissues. If I want to cleanse the tissues, I must also be willing to cleanse the issues that live there. So I add emotional cleansing and radical self love to my cleansing ritual. Although I may be more scared to go there, the more I release, the more amazing my life will get. So I dive deep into the depths of my soul. I will be grateful I did. I trust myself.

I SET MY INTENTIONS HERE...

1. My intention for this cleanse is?
2. I know I will be successful when?
3. I want to lose weight? Look younger? Have more energy? Heal my body? Think clearer? Feel happier? Feel sexier?
4. How I want to feel in my body is?
5. How I want to feel in my life is?
6. I commit to release __?__ habit, as it no longer serves me.
7. Three actions I will take to release this habit are?
8. One person I am forgiving is?
9. Three actions I will take to forgive this person are?
10. One thought that I keep thinking about myself that is not empowering me is?
11. The new empowering thought that will replace this old disempowering one is?
12. A dream I wish to fulfill is __?__
13. Three actions I will take towards this dream are?

CHAPTER 15

SUPER CLEANSING TECHNIQUES

LET'S TALK ABOUT TOXINS and most importantly how to get them out of my body as quickly and easily as possible. When my body knows it is cleansing, it will begin releasing toxins that it has safely tucked away inside my cells for my protection. These toxins will now be in my blood stream, making their way down to my bowel and onto my tongue. I might feel sick or nauseous if I allow these toxins to swim around in my blood for too long. So I get them out fast. The faster I can get rid of my toxins, the better I feel.

My body is always trying to heal me and cleanse me. When I stop ingesting toxins, the body works much harder and faster to push the overload out. So I help my body to take all my crap out faster. I will take my JUICY cleanse to the next level and get rid of my toxins faster by adding in saunas, enemas, colonics, proper pooping techniques, water purification, body scrubbing and mouth cleansing.

A more detailed description of mouth cleansing, proper bowel care, enemas and colonics is in the following chapters, so for now, this is an overview.

Infrared saunas, dry saunas, steam saunas and hot springs are a great way to detox and get the gunk out through my skin. Skin is my biggest elimination organ and is a super highway for crap coming in and also crap coming out. I use my skin to help me get the crap out. Unlike other saunas, infrared saunas heat me from the inside out, so their effects are much faster and more powerful. A few times throughout my JUICY cleanse, I have a 20 to 30 minute sauna session. I allow the high heat to sweat the toxins out of me. I will try using essential oils and rubbing them on my hands, breathing them in and spraying them inside the sauna to help cleanse my lungs and open up my nasal passageways. *DoTerra* or *Young Living* essential oils are the purest.

Hot natural thermal springs are much healthier than hot tubs. Hot tubs are full of chlorine, which is a toxin for my body and gets absorbed into my skin as I soak. Natural thermal springs have minerals and healing properties in the water and have been used for centuries in treating people's health problems. It is healthy and very beneficial for me to spend a day soaking in thermal springs. My body will absorb minerals through my skin and also help me alkaline my body. A lot of mineral spring pools will also have mineral drinking water to help heal my insides. I drink this healing water.

- - ♡ - -

Waterfalls, Oceans, Rivers and Water Temples are also an amazing way to cleanse my body and my emotional state. The ocean is full of salty magnesium which is a much needed mineral for my body. Swimming in the ocean allows me to absorb this mineral through my skin. Magnesium calms my body, relieves the nervous system and activates the spark of life inside me. So ocean time is a super healing time. Natural waters also help me wash off the unwanted negative energies, EMF radiation from cell phones and cell towers, invigorate my body cells and charge up my system with the power of nature.

Dipping in or rinsing off with water during my cleanse allows me an opportunity to release all that is no longer serving me through the cleansing power of water. Every shower or bath can now become a cleansing and releasing ritual. The water will happily help me release my crap. Also I start drinking natural raw spring water and look for a spring near me.

Colonics and Enemas are amazing ways to get the excess fecal matter and toxins out of my body fast. They are water irrigation inside my colon. Colonics are administered by a colon hydro therapist and enemas I can do on my own. Both are safe and can really help me. Enemas used to be administered as part of the homeopathic natural medicine that was practiced. Homeopathic doctors would come to people's house and if their body was in fever or ill, they would give them an enema to release the toxins.

A fever happens when the body gets overloaded with toxins and can't heal itself fast enough. The body heats up in an attempt to sweat the toxins out of the body. An enema will flush the toxins out of my bowel to release them out of my body.

Dry Brushing is a way to open my skin pours so the toxins can be released through my skin, which is my biggest elimination organ. Dry brushing is done with a firm bristle brush on my dry skin. It is best to do dry brushing outside or in the bathroom, as dead skin cells will be flying off of me. It is more effective to brush my skin when I am dry then wet in the shower. Yet it is also very effective to scrub my skin in the shower with a brush or rough face cloth. When I open up my skin pores, I create an open doorway for my toxins to come out. Scrubbing my skin will also help me look younger with softer skin as I have scuffed off all the old dead stuff.

Mouth Cleansing first thing in the morning is super important, as all my toxins are sitting on my tongue when I wake up. My body works all night to clean house and pushes the toxins to my tongue and my bowel to be released in the morning. So I make sure I clean my mouth before I drink anything so I am not swallowing the toxins back down.

I make bathroom switches and stop putting toxic creams, lotions and perfumes on my skin because within 20 minutes they are swimming in my bloodstream. Anything I put on my skin is like I have eaten it. I switch to a good quality coconut oil, the same kind I would use for cooking, for my new skin lotion. It works awesome and is easily absorbed into my skin so I won't feel greasy. I start switching to using real essential oils as my perfumes and start adding them to my medicine cabinet as my medicine. I throw out the toxic pharmaceutical creams, lotions, pills, quick fix medicines and start concentrating on healing my body from the inside out. I start using natural make up, shampoos, conditioners, soaps, toothpaste, face cleansers and mouth washes. When I stop ingesting the toxins, my body will be much happier and able to heal me quicker. There is no room in my JUICY lifestyle for a toxic bathroom cabinet or shower stall.

I cleanse my bathroom at the same time as I cleanse myself. Most likely my bathroom is filled with toxic lotions and potions, so I throw them out! Now loving my body and myself so much more, I will no longer poison my body with toxic pharmaceuticals and products.

ISSUES LIVE IN MY TISSUES
I AM WILLING TO CLEANSE THEM OUT
I AM WILLING TO LET THEM GO
I AM MORE FREE & MORE HAPPY

- - ♡ - -

CHAPTER 16

TIME TO HAVE
A KISSABLE MOUTH

M Y BODY IS WORKING TO GET TOXINS out of my body all the time, day and night. When I sleep, my body soldiers sweep up toxins and push them to the exit points of my body for morning garbage removal.

The two exit points are my BOWEL and my MOUTH! Every night my body has a cleansing PARTY and when it is over, the toxins are lined up at the exit doors ready to leave. So I let them out!

I will learn several ways to clean my bowel in the upcoming chapters, so now I learn how to clean my mouth, especially my tongue.

From now on and for the rest of my life, I take on the practice to clean my mouth every morning before I eat food or drink any liquids. If I don't, then I am swallowing the toxic party guests back down and wasting all the cleaning work my body did all night.

On my JUICY food cleanse, I may notice that my tongue looks extra yucky with white muck all over it and my breath might become extra stinky. This is because my body is cleaning much more rigorously during my cleanse and placing all the toxic waste on my tongue waiting for me to clean it. During my JUICY cleanse, toxins will want to be released out of my body, so I make sure I clean my tongue first thing in the morning. Then after my cleanse and as I continue my new JUICY lifestyle, I will continue cleaning my tongue and my mouth every morning before I swallow anything down.

The health of my mouth and my teeth are indicators of the health of my body. If my teeth are yellow, rotting and my gums are inflamed then I do something about it. My smile is an important part of me and my mouth speaks my truth, so I allow this area to be radiant. If I feel embarrassed about my teeth or my mouth health, then I will reduce the expression I give to the world. So I clean my mouth. I whiten my teeth naturally. I freshen my breath. I allow my mouth to radiate my health.

Starting right now, I get the toxins out. I clean my mouth, I have fresh breath, I create stronger gums and whiter teeth, I prevent teeth rot and cavities, My mouth will feel so fresh and clean, and I will feel happier in my heart.

AMAZING TIPS FOR CLEANING MY MOUTH....

1. BRUSH WITH HEALTHIER TOOTHPASTE – I stop
    using fluoride toothpastes and switch to an all natural brand.
    I have been brainwashed that I need to ingest this toxic
    chemical called fluoride that workers wear hasmat suits to
    touch.   Fluoride calcifies my pineal gland, which allows
    me to connect to my sovereignty and intuition.   Flouride
    was put into our water supply first by Hitler to make a
    docile population. When my pineal gland is calcified, I will
    become a follower who doesn't question the system instead
    of a leader who speaks up. I start using a natural toothpaste
    and I also start SPEAKING UP!

2. SCRAPE MY TONGUE - My tongue is full of toxins
    every morning so I use my tooth brush or a tongue scraper
    to scrape my tongue.   The cleaner my tongue, the more
    my taste buds will awaken and my ability to taste even the
    tiniest details will be expanded. If I currently eat processed
    food, then my taste buds are numbed out.   As I cleanse
    my body and my tongue, I will notice my new heightened
    ability to taste every detail.

3. START OIL PULLING - Oil pulling is an ancient
    practice used for centuries and an awesome way to cleanse
    my mouth of all the toxins first thing in the morning. I
    swig a small amount of food grade coconut oil or untoasted
    sesame oil into my mouth upon waking and swish it around
    for 5-10 minutes. The oil gets in between my teeth and
    gums, and grabs all the toxins so I can spit them out. I can
    putter around my house, tidy up, get myself ready, go to

the bathroom, do what I need as I swish the oil around in my mouth. I do not have to stand in front of the mirror to do this. It is much easier to multi task getting things done swishing my oil at the same time. I then spit the oil into a garbage can. I will notice how clean my mouth feels and how smooth my teeth feel. Oil pulling will get into all the areas between my teeth to clean the germs and will also help heal my gums. I will notice my teeth getting whiter and whiter. I don't spit my coconut oil down the sink as it can harden in cold climates and plug up my sink.

OIL PULL RECIPE

Use: untoasted sesame or food grade coconut oil
Take a swig of oil first thing in the morning
Swoosh it around all my teeth, gums, tongue
Keep it going for 5-10 minutes
Spit it out into a garbage can or outside
Not down the sink

4. FLOSS MY TEETH – I get a natural dental floss and I use it. Most food and germs are lodged in between my teeth and my toothbrush can't get them, so I floss them out. I floss daily as part of my new JUICY lifestyle ritual. Sometimes I forget or get lazy and that is ok, I keep my floss visible so I remember. I can take my flossing to the next level and place a drop of essential oil on my finger and run the floss string through the oil. I try *DoTerra* On Guard or Oregano essential oil as they are safe to ingest. This is an easy way to get more medicine between my teeth

and on my gums. I can also use other healing tinctures or medicinal mixtures to coat my dental floss with. I try what works for me. *Young Living* is another brand of edible essential oils.

5. USE PETRA'S INCREDIBLE MOUTH WASH - Just like the oil pulling this mouth wash will get into all the cracks and little areas that my toothbrush can not. It foams up inside my mouth as the mouthwash eats away all my mouth bacteria.

PETRA'S FABULOUS MOUTH WASH RECIPE

3% food grade hydrogen peroxide
Clean drinking water
1-2 drops edible essential oil *DoTerra* Peppermint

In glass jar or water bottle, combine the above
1 part hydrogen peroxide to 2 parts water
Add few drops essential oil
Take a swig and swoosh it around
Keep in for a few seconds, it will get bubbly like champagne
Spit out into the sink

If it hurts my teeth a little – then I dilute the mixture with a little more water. If my mixture is too strong, then I will feel an ache in my teeth nerves, so I add more water.

Food grade hydrogen peroxide is safe if swallowed and is alkaline. I don't swallow it but know that it is safe to put into my mouth. It is used in cancer healing as a quick way to alkaline the body. I will research this method of healing if I am interested. It is an in depth system not explained in this book.

I am not swallowing this mouth wash. I am swooshing it around inside my mouth and just like oil pulling, I spit it out. My mouth will feel super fresh and clean. My teeth will keep getting whiter and whiter, and my gums healthier.

A LOVE NOTE FROM PETRA: I use this mouthwash in the morning upon waking and throughout the day. I keep a container in my car and in my office. I use it to cleanse and freshen my mouth all the time and I love it!!! I used to oil pull for a long time, then changed it up with this mouth wash. I still oil pull at times, yet have found this to be my new favorite thing. Try both and see which one you prefer.

- - ♡ - -

6. REMOVE MY MERCURY FILLINGS - If I have mercury fillings then I get them removed from a professional holistic dentist as soon as possible. My health and I are worth it. Mercury is one of the most poisonous substances on our planet yet the dental association continue to claim its safety and continue putting it inside people's mouths. This is ridiculous! I can do more research on mercury fillings and the harm they cause my body system without me realizing

it. Mercury fillings are always off gassing especially when I drink hot or cold drinks. When I kiss someone with mercury fillings, I am sharing mercury off gassing vapors with them. Many people claim expedited healing in their body when they remove the mercury. Major illnesses like alzheimer's, autism, fibromyalgia, MS, Parkinson's, Crohn's, digestive issues and many more are linked to mercury in the body and have been proven to shift once fillings are removed. Once I have remove my fillings, I will do a rigorous JUICY cleanse with saunas, colonics, chlorella, charcoal, etc to get rid of the excess mercury living in my body.

A LOVE NOTE FROM PETRA: I had my mercury fillings removed about 10 years ago and did a rigorous cleansing regime after the procedure. I did lots of colonics and infrared saunas. I drank lots of chlorella as it takes metals out of the system and ate lots of cilantro, which removes metals also. I drank activated charcoal drinks and flushed my body with liquids. Since I didn't have any major health issues prior and was already on the cleansing path, I didn't notice any major body differences. I do, however, feel such a sense of peace within that I do not have toxic mercury in my body any longer. I also got all my respective kissing partners to remove their mercury fillings for their health and the health of our kissing time. So please take this extra cleansing regime on and get rid of the TOXIC mercury out of your system and have your fillings replaced. You are worth it!

IT IS MY BIRTHRIGHT TO BE HEALTHY

MY BODY LOVES ME

I LOVE ME

I AM BRAVE AND I CLEANSE MY BODY

I AM HEALHTY AND FULL OF ENERGY

- - ♡ - -

CHAPTER 17

WHAT COLOR IS MY TONGUE?

MY TONGUE IS MY WINDOW TO MY INSIDES. My tongue is a spongy organ that will show me the state of my health and mirror to me what my internal system looks like. Chinese medicine uses the tongue as an indicator of a person's health and much can be read on the tongue. So what color is my tongue?

My tongue may look 'normal' or it may already look white, yellow or grey. Once I start cleansing, I will see my tongue transform. So I watch my tongue. As my cells start releasing stored up toxins, my tongue will change colors. It will change to white, grey, yellow and look absolutely disgusting. Kissing someone is just not a good idea during my JUICY cleanse, until I clear up my insides. There might be a thick coating that forms on my tongue and it might actually look hairy. I will be able to gauge the depth of my toxic body and the cleansing that is occurring just by watching my tongue.

I remember to tongue scrape and clean my mouth as often as possible to continue releasing this stored up toxic matter. As I clean my insides and my tongue, my taste buds will clean too and I will be able to taste in more detail. I now have a greater appreciation for my spongy tongue organ and the wisdom it provides for me. I work with my body to clean it so I live a longer, healthier, more vibrant life.

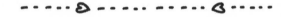

CHAPTER 18

PROPER POOPING

L ET'S TALK ABOUT A SIMPLE POOPING TECHNIQUE that will cleanse and heal me every time I go to the bathroom, which should be every day or a few times a day.

From NOW on and for the REST of my life, I start propping my feet up on a stepping stool or on my bathroom garbage can when I poo. The modern toilet has made us all SICK. Our bodies were never designed to poo sitting up right, we were designed to SQUAT. When I prop my feet up, I replicate the squatting position.

Propping my feet up, opens up my bowel passage ways and my poo comes out easily and effortlessly. When I sit on the toilet up right with my feet on the floor, my poo has a harder time coming out. I might push, feel constipated or struggle to get poo out of my system. Constipation is the #1 sickness plaguing the whole world. Most people are constipated or carrying around excess fecal matter that they have a hard time releasing. This blocked system is making us all sick. When my body is not clean on the inside, it will create sickness somewhere else in my system. My poo is the waste byproduct of my body computer machine and the garbage needs to keep coming out for me to be healthy. I have to get the garbage out of my system or it will pollute my system.

Imagine I am living in a house and I use 1 bedroom to store all my garbage. My old food, kitchen waste, snotty tissues, used toilet paper and anything else I would normally throw away. Now imagine after a few weeks, a few months, a few years this toxic waste dump in my bedroom becomes stinky, rotting, fermenting and putrefying. It attracts rodents, bugs and germs. I can smell and sense my rotting bedroom garbage all the time. The smell is now polluting every other room in my house. It is making me uncomfortable to live in my house. It is making me feel awkward to invite my friends over. It is making my life not FUN and not HAPPY.

YES! This is the same with my body. All of that old undigested food, environmental chemicals, food colorings, old dead cells and putrefying hard to digest meat are polluting every organ and section of my body. This old waste I am carrying around is making my health and my life much less FUN and much less HAPPY!

My bowel is the king to my entire system. If it is plugged and full, it will affect the rest of my body, all other organs and my entire body system. Cleansing my bowel is the fastest way for me to heal and feel better.

My digestive system is like a long curly waterslide. Food enters the mouth and slides down my digestive track waterslide twisting and turning for about 8.5 meters (28 feet), before it gets flushed into my bowel swimming pool. With so much food and chemicals sliding down the waterslide, eventually my swimming pool gets dirty and I have to clean it. Unfortunately a few poos a week will not be enough to fully clean my swimming pool, so flushing my system with juices and healing liquids is the only way I can fully clean my bowel.

I might feel embarrassed talking about or reading about poo. Yet the truth is, I POO and it is an essential body function of all species on the planet. So instead of sitting on the toilet for hours in constipated frustration, I start drinking green juices, green smoothies and I start using my pooping stool to heal my body and get rid of constipation forever!!!

If I have a beer belly or excess fat around my mid-drift, I most likely have an enlarged inflamed unhealthy colon that has excess fecal matter in it. My colon is on fire and it is asking for my help. My colon will enlarge to carry what is inside. The more I put in, the more my colon will grow to accommodate its contents. The more unhealthy and agitated my colon is, the more inflamed it will be. An inflamed colon is puffy, throbbing and on fire. In order to heal my colon, I have to remove the garbage, stop agitating it with acidic food and acidic thoughts, and start eating and drinking food that will take my inflammation down.

Even if I am a skinny person, I will be surprised how much poo I have in my system once I start flushing out my digestive track. 50% of my poo is food and the other 50% is dead cells that are constantly dying off in every second. So even if I am pooping every day, it might not be enough to get rid of all the waste my body is accumulating. Over time my poo gets lodged into little crevasses and little pockets that are created in my digestive track. Poo also gets stuck on my microvilli, which are tiny hair like projections in my small intestine that help absorb all the nutrients into my system. When they are covered with hard old poo, they cannot do their work and my body can no longer absorbs any nutrients.

This JUICY food cleanse will help me flush out my colon, small intestine, large intestine, gut and clean my microvilli. As I drink daily juices and smoothies my intestinal track and bowel will release excess fecal matter hiding in every corner of my system. I will start using a pooping stool to really transform my world. I will poo easily, effortlessly and eliminate constipation out of my life forever.

A LOVE NOTE FROM PETRA: My clients and I do enemas and colonics during our JUICY cleanses. I have added coffee enemas into my lifestyle as a monthly regime or when ever I feel my body needs it. All of my juicing clients, who are not eating anything solid for days or weeks, are always shocked as to what comes out of them. Once you get focused on cleansing your bowel, you too will be shocked how much excess fecal matter you have inside of you. I love talking about this important, yet uncomfortable for some, topic. Happy to bring it out into the open, so you can fully understand your body and not feel embarrassed to do enemas or colonics to release your excess fecal matter. I encourage you to try out this ancient way of healing the body naturally. Your doctor will most likely not understand or try to discourage you from cleansing your bowel. They would rather give you creams and pills that they get commissions from. Yet the ancient way of healing patients was to heal with enemas, administered by homeopathic doctors. Healing through toxic waste removal makes sense once you understand the body and how it heals itself. It is my intent that through reading this book, you understand how your body works so you can finally take your health into your hands. It is time!

- - ♥ - -

I STOP CARRYING AROUND EXTRA
CRAP IN MY BODY
I GET RID OF MY POO
I STOP HANGING ON TO IT
IT IS MAKING ME SICK
IT IS MAKING MY BODY TOXIC
I LET GO
I LET IT ALL GO

- - ♡ - -

CHAPTER 19

LET'S DO ENEMAS

D URING MY JUICY FOOD CLEANSE, I focuss on getting the toxins out of my body as fast as possible and getting rid of any excess fecal matter that I might be carrying around.

Drinking lots of liquids, juices, water, smoothies and eating more raw foods full of liquid, oxygen and fiber will help me poo a lot more. This JUICY food cleanse will help me scrape my intestines so I get more fecal matter out faster.

ENEMAS are a GREAT way to flush my colon and release toxins out fast. Before modern allopathic medicine, medicine was homeopathic, natural and more connected to the natural workings of the body. The first thing that homeopathic doctors prescribed when a person was sick or had fever was an enema. No, not pharmaceutical pills to suppress the symptoms but an enema to release the toxins out of the body that might be causing the body harm.

Homeopathic doctors knew that the body, in fever or in toxic state, is like a volcano, hot and ready to explode. By doing an enema, the toxins are released fast, resulting in the body volcano calming down and becoming dormant again.

When the toxic load gets too much and my body can't release fast enough, my body goes into toxic shock and a fever kicks in. The fever is my body's way of wanting to push all the toxins out of my body as fast as possible through the biggest elimination organ, my skin.

So by doing an enema, I release the toxic build up in my body and release the pressure. The body can relax and continue its healing process. Its like my sink drain is plugged and doing an enema releases the clog in my pipes.

I can do enemas at home on my own. It might feel strange at first or I might be nervous. I don't allow myself to worry. It is painless, quite easy and provides so many healing benefits.

- Do an enema when I am feeling a cold coming on

- Do an enema when I had a night of drinking and heavy eating the night before

- Do an enema while I am JUICY cleansing to increase the power of the cleanse

- Do an enema to youthen my body and release years of stored up waste

I can buy enema bags at some health food stores or buy online on Amazon and they are inexpensive. So I get one and I TRY IT!

I can do 2 kinds of enemas – luke warm water or luke warm coffee. I use ONLY filtered CLEAN WATER and I use only ORGANIC COFFEE, since this is going into my blood stream. I want to avoid chemicals, fluoride, chlorine and toxins found in tap water and sprayed on regular coffee.

HOW TO DO AN ENEMA...

1. Clamp the enema bag hose with the provided clip and fill the enema bag with my luke warm water or my specifically made coffee mixture.

2. Remove the blue plastic hose cover and lubricate the end of the hose with coconut oil or olive oil.

3. Either place towels on the floor for me to lay on or fill my tub with hot water and soak while doing the enema. Petra prefers laying in a warm bathtub.

4. Hang enema bag on shower head or towel rack, somewhere to elevate it a few feet above my body.

5. Squat to insert the hose into my bum gently and slowly till it goes a few inches in. The hose is really thin and I barely feel it.

6. Lay on my back and get comfortable.

7. Breathe. I am ok, this is painless.

8. Release the hose clamp and slowly start filling my body with the water or coffee mixture.

9. I might need to put the clamp back on to stop the liquid flow and do this in stages. Breathe. Relax. Then release the rest of the enema bag in. Take my time and listen to my body. During this process, I rub my belly or jiggle it to help move the mixture in. This also helps prevent any cramping and eases the liquid in easier.

10. Ideally I hold the water or coffee for 11 minutes. Set a timer or have my phone handy so I can check the time.

11. Meditate, breathe, visualize releasing the mental and physical crap out of my body. Chant the mantra, "I release, I let go" over and over again.

12. Massage my belly and digestive track. Push the energy from my right side to my left side. Jiggle my belly with my hands to move the water in and move the stuff out. Massaging makes it easier to hang on to the enema mixture and helps loosen up my fecal matter.

13. When ready, get up, go to toilet and release using pooping stool.

14. If I need to get up and go to the toilet before the 11 minutes, do it. Resist the urge to do so by breathing and rubbing my belly. At the same time, honor my body and be gentle with myself. If I have to release, then I release.

MORE ENEMA TIPS...

1. The first few times I do an enema, I might not be able to hold for 11 minutes. I might feel cramps and need to release. It is ok. I listen to my body and I also don't stop at the first sign of a little discomfort. I get centered in my mind, focus and breathe.

2. Most importantly I listen to my body.

3. I can also put in ½ the enema bag mixture and see how I feel. I may need to go quickly to the bathroom, so I get up to poo. Then I get back into the bathtub, insert the hose back into my bum and allow in the other ½ of the enema mixture. Most likely I will be able to hold the other ½ much longer. When the poo is right there and ready to come out, it's better I let it out and then do a second round.

4. After I am finished, wash enema bag for next use. Clean hose end with soap or hydrogen peroxide.

5. Never lose my enema bag clamp, as it is the most important piece and without it my enema bag will not work.

6. During my JUICY food cleanse, I do enemas daily or every other day. If I am starting a JUICY lifestyle then I do enemas once per week and then once per month to get my system cleaner.

7. I will be releasing toxins and excess fecal matter from my bowel, and also stimulating my liver for cleansing.

8. If the coffee or water enema remains inside and nothing comes out into the toilet, that is ok, it means I am very dehydrated.

9. Do my enema after I have had a bowel movement so I can hold the liquid in longer. If I am not having bowel movements often, then I do an enema RIGHT AWAY!

10. If the coffee enema makes me jittery, then dilute the coffee mixture even more.

11. The enema might lower my blood pressure. If so, eat something before or after, like 1/2 banana or a fruitier fresh juice. I am ok.

12. Added benefits of enemas are energy, clarity and vitality.

13. Coffee enemas are one of the greatest ways to flush toxins out of my body and cleanse my liver as the coffee starts to pump the liver and bile is released.

14. Healing and detox centers all over the world are using enemas and colonics to heal people of all major illnesses including cancer. Most do daily coffee enemas for weeks.

15. I might feel nervous to do my FIRST one and I DO IT anyway. I will see how easy it actually is and how great I feel.

16. I might prefer doing my enema in the evening, more than the morning because I may want to relax and lie down after. Although sometimes a late night coffee enema can keep me awake as the coffee goes into my blood stream and can stimulate me.

17. Do an enema if I feel bloated and my belly doesn't feel good. This can help me quickly, especially if I have plans to go out and am just not feeling so great. An enema will help me release the gas in my colon, so I feel more comfortable to put on my jeans and head out the house.

18. Enemas have been used since ancient times by homeopathic doctors. It is only our current medical system that is not open to them and most doctors will discourage me from doing them and from doing colonics. Most doctors are not versed in making me well as they are in making me dependent on pills. So I take my health into my hands and do what feels right for me.

WARM COFFEE ENEMA RECIPE - ONE TIME USE

2 Tbsp. organic coffee
6 cups filtered or spring water

Place in sauce pan and bring to boil
Boil for 10 min and let cool with a finger test
Pour through a fine mesh strainer or nut mylk bag
to strain grinds
Pour into mason jar to store or into enema bag to use

MY BOWEL IS THE KING
TO MY ENTIRE SYSTEM
I CLEAN MY BOWEL
I LET GO OF THE OLD CRAP
I AM CLEAN
MY BOWEL IS HAPPY

- - ♡ - -

CHAPTER 20

LET'S DO COLONICS

OLONICS ARE THE NEXT LEVEL OF ENEMAS. Enemas I can do myself at home and colonics I go to a colonic center and a Colon Hydro Therapist does the colonic for me.

Colonics are treatments that wash my colon through water irrigation. They put about 5 gallons of water through my colon and really help wash me out. They are easy, painless and impactful.

I always take good quality probiotics when doing colonics and enemas to make sure my gut flora stays healthy. The water coming up inside my system can take good bacteria with it, so I want to add the good bacteria back in with probiotics, kefirs and fermented healthy food during colon cleansing.

Even if I am doing a gentler cleanse like cutting out meat or dairy for a month, colonics are still a good way to add in extra cleansing power. However they do work better when I am eating a diet that supports the CLEANING and FLUSHING of the internal system. I take full advantage of this powerful cleansing technique and flush my digestive track first with JUICY liquids, so I can help get more garbage out.

On my JUICY food cleanse, I add in colonics. As I drink, I will be scraping a lot of old crap off my intestinal walls and I want that stuff out of my body FAST. On a 7 day liquid cleanse, I do 3 colonic sessions spaced out every 2 days.

Colonics can feel like an evasive process especially since someone is there with me. I might feel afraid that poo will fly everywhere and I will be super embarrassed, but it's actually quite a clean and sterile process.

The first session usually loosens most of my inside crap. The second session seems to get a lot more out. The third session continues to get more out. After my third session, I will know if I need a fourth session. My Colon Hydro Therapist can help me gauge this as well. If I am releasing a lot, then I go for a fourth session to keep the cleaning going.

The most important process of doing these colonics is my willingness to let my crap go. Without realizing it, I can hang on energetically to my emotions, pains, hurts and the garbage in my system that even the colonic cannot release it. I could have a colonic session where nothing comes out. It is possible I am squeaky clean or, most likely, I am emotionally unable to let go. My emotional state is holding on to my physical and mental crap and I have to be willing to let it go. I lie on the colonic table and repeat the mantra, "I release. I let go what is no longer serving me. I let this crap go. I release. I let go."

Colon is the king to my entire body system. My colon is connected to every organ and system in my body. When it is cleaned and running optimally again, the rest of my body responds and feels this healing. When the colon is toxic and full of excess sludge, the rest of my organs are affected and sickness sets in.

WHAT WILL COLONICS DO FOR MY COLON?

1. HEAL MY COLON - Toxins that have built up over time are gently removed from my colon in a series of treatments so my colon can operate again, like it's supposed to. This is a colon rejuvenation treatment.

2. EXERCISE MY COLON - Toxins weaken my colon and ruin its proper functioning. The gentle filling and releasing of the water activates the muscles and exercises them. A great workout for my colon.

3. RESHAPE MY COLON - When problems or excess fecal matter live in my colon for too long, they reshape the colon. The colon is a muscle so it enlarges when it is full and contracts when it is empty. If my colon is full of poo for a long period of time, the muscle stretches and changes shape. The water therapy along with the massaging of my tummy by the Colon Hydro Therapist will help eliminate

bulging pockets of poop and narrowed spastic constrictions. My colon can get back to its natural state.

4. HYDRATION - Water is absorbed into my body through the colon and this helps flush out my toxins faster. Circulation of my blood is increased resulting in greater bathing of my cells. When my cells are cleaned and running optimally, my body is healthy. If my cells are not functioning properly then major disease is the result. If my cells are full of toxins, then my body is puffy and toxic. Having a healthy working colon means hydration is filtered through my whole body to hydrate and flush out each of my cells.

MORE COLONIC TIPS...

1. During my 7 day JUICY food cleanse, I do 3 or 4 colonics. One every 2 or 3 days.

2. Example 3 colonics every other day:

    First session - loosens the old hard caked on poo that is glued to the walls of my intestines and colon. Even if I poo every day, I probably have old stuff lining my walls.

    Second session - releases the loosened up stuff from the first session and from all my JUICY flushing. As my Hydro Therapist massages my tummy, she is helping push and move old hard stuff along my intestinal track to be released out.

Third session - releases more loosened stuff. Usually not as much stuff is coming out, but if I notice a lot of poo and mucous coming out, then I will consider a 4th and 5th session. My Hydro Therapist will help advise me. If I continue releasing and having major releases, then YIPEEEE and I keep my colonic sessions going. Stuff has loosened, so I help my body let it go. I can't afford to carry the crap around with me any longer, so I allow myself to release it all.

3. It is possible that I have tape worms or parasites in my body as most people do. Ideally my JUICY flushing and my colonic sessions will get them out. If I am a meat eater, it is likely I have parasites inside me transferred via my meat. I drink diatomaceous earth super cleanser water (recipe in the upcoming chapters) to kill parasites internally during my JUICY cleanse, so I have an opportunity to flush them out during my colonic sessions.

4. Colon Hydrotherapy sessions cost about $60 - $80 per session and sometimes I can get package deals. It's an investment in myself and in my health. Enemas are much cheaper and very effective also, but not quite as powerful as a colonic. I choose which feels more right for me. Ideally I do both during my JUICY cleanse and new JUICY lifestyle.

5. Find a Therapist that I feel comfortable with and that is knowledgeable. This is an intimate experience so I want to make sure I feel good and safe. Make sure they massage

my belly and help move the old hard poo out. I ask for support, this is my session and I am worth it.

6. Take very good quality probiotics after my session. Water irrigation does affect my gut flora (bacteria), so it's important I help my gut flora get back to an optimal healthy state. I can buy probiotics at health food stores or healthy grocery stores. Found usually in the fridge section.

7. I can have my eyes closed during my colonic session or I can watch the whole process. I might want to see what "crap" is coming out of my body, so I watch the clear tube to see what is coming through.

8. Drink warm tea, soup or something soothing after my colonic and take my probiotics. It feels good to have something comforting in my belly after a colonic.

9. I might feel a bit tired after my colonic so I schedule them in the latter part of my day so I can go home to rest. It's possible I will feel super energized too. Everyone reacts differently.

10. If I am adding saunas into my JUICY cleanse, then I do them right after my colonic as this feels relaxing for me. This is self love, so I do what feels right for me.

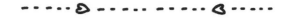

CHAPTER 21

SUPER CLEANSERS

HERE IS A LIST OF SUPER CLEANSERS I can add to my JUICY cleanse and my JUICY lifestyle if I want to take things to the next level.

1. PROBIOTICS – good gut flora, one of most important supplements to balance the insides

2. ACTIVATED CHARCOAL – pulls all toxins out of body, super alkaline, helps me poo

3. MAGNESIUM – oxygenates colon, helps me poo, much needed mineral for the body

4. FOOD GRADE DIATOMACEOUS EARTH – high silica, colon cleanser, detoxifier, kills parasites

5. BENTONITE CLAY – alkaline, pulls toxins out of the body, eat and put into bath

6. PSYLLIUM HUSK – fiber scrapes me out, binds and pulls the toxins out of body

7. ALOE VERA GEL – soothing for the digestive track, takes inflammation down, great for skin

8. TURMERIC CURCUMIN – need black pepper to activate, major anti inflammatory, cancer healer

9. HEMP CBD OIL – major anti inflammatory, massive healing in body, supports nervous system, helps heart heal

10. CHLORELLA – pulls heavy metals out of body, chlorophyll boost, super protein

11. SPIRULINA – chlorophyll boost, super protein, power green

12. WHEATGRASS – major alkalizer, detoxifier, chlorophyll boost, super protein

When I am using these super cleansers, it is important I drink lots of water and liquids to flush out the toxins that they are binding to. The cleansers will do their job and grab the toxins, but I need to help flush everything out of my body.

1. PROBIOTICS

My gut has good and bad bacteria inside. When I eat crappy food, drink alcohol, eat lots of sugar, think stress and drink chlorine fluoride tap water, then the bad bacteria inside me grows bigger and takes over my gut. An over growth of bad bacteria can eventually cause me gut issues, constipation, skin issues, brain fogginess, yeast infections, candida and is at the stem of cancer and other major dis-eases of the body.

Probiotics are high doses of good bacteria in pill form. When I eat a healthier diet, cleanse and add in probiotics, I help the good bacteria grow again in my gut. The bad bacteria gets smaller, the good bacteria gets bigger and my body gets back into balance.

When I do colonics and enemas, I am lightly disturbing the gut flora and it is important that I supplement with high quality probiotics to keep my gut balanced.

I START RIGHT NOW....I go buy a really good quality and high dose brand. I take it for a month or a few months to rebalance my gut flora and get my body back into alignment. The faster my gut is healthy, the faster my entire system is thriving again.

HOW TO EAT: Swallow a few pills on an empty stomach in the morning and through out the day, depending on my dosage and how quickly I need to heal my gut.

Probiotics are also found in fermented foods like raw sauerkraut, raw kimchi, raw apple cider vinegar, coconut yogurt and coconut kefir. I add these foods in as part of my new JUICY lifestyle.

2. ACTIVATED CHARCOAL

Different from the charcoal pills given in conventional medical system. Activated charcoal is made from coconut husks, hemp stalks or bamboo branches. It is created in a closed high heat oven to create activated charcoal that is full of activated minerals and good bacteria to help alkaline my body. Charcoal binds to toxins in my body and pulls them out. It scrapes my insides and helps my colon release stored up fecal matter. It is said to help over 10,000 various ailments of the body. It will help me poo, alkaline my body and detoxify me much faster.

HOW TO EAT: Mix ½ teaspoon in water and drink. Use a jar to shake the mixture to blend it better. It tastes neutral, a little like drinking gritty water and is easy to consume as part of my JUICY cleanse or throughout my new JUICY lifestyle. If my tummy is feeling off or I feel acidic, I can drink a glass of charcoal water for instant relief. Drink lots of extra water when drinking charcoal.

3. MAGNESIUM

This mineral is needed for my body and all its neurological function. It is the spark of life in my body and needed for all my joints and muscles to feel flexible and happy. Magnesium stops being produced by my body after the age of 30 and so adding it in as a supplement is very healthy. There are 2 kinds of magnesium I can buy. One oxygenates my colon, so it helps me poo and can also be used as a powerful cleansing agent. The other bypasses my colon and goes straight into my bloodstream. Both relax my muscles, help ease me into rest and sleep better. This mineral is needed for my body to function optimally.

Magnesium is also found in raw chocolate, the ocean and some spring water. I can buy pure magnesium salt for my bath and magnesium oil spray to absorb via my skin. Epsom salts are a processed version of magnesium and are still quite effective in relaxing my body and removing all the negative ions of me. The ocean is full of this powerful magnesium salt, so I soak in the ocean as much as I can.

HOW TO EAT: Buy in pill form with various levels of potency (from 400 mg to 2000 mg) or a flavored powder that I mix in water. Eat raw chocolate or drink raw chocolate. Swim in the ocean or soak in Epsom salt baths. Buy magnesium oil and spray it on my body to be absorbed via my skin.

A LOVE NOTE FROM PETRA: My favorite way to eat magnesium is via raw chocolate and I believe that when we crave chocolate, it is actually magnesium that our body desires. So eating chocolate is healthy as long as it is raw and not processed. Avoid soy, dairy, white sugar, oils and artificial fillers when you buy chocolate. Buy it at a healthier grocery store, read the ingredients and ideally buy it raw. Or make your own and I love teaching how to do that. I am a great chocolate maker!!!

4. FOOD GRADE DIATOMACEOUS EARTH

A great cleanser, binder to toxins to help pull them out of my body and parasite killer. On a microscopic level, diatomaceous earth is shards of glass. When these shards are ingested by parasites or worms in my body, it rips their bellies and they die. Buy the food grade brand found in health food stores and not the garden kind found hardware stores. It tastes like dirt water and is quite flavorless. It is easy to drink. It is also great for growing strong hair, skin and nails as it is silica. The garden kind is used to naturally kill slugs and other critters when I sprinkle it around my garden vegetables.

HOW TO EAT: Mix 1 teaspoon of earth in water and drink. Tastes like chalky water.

5. BENTONITE CLAY

Since ancient times clays have been used as an external and internal cleanser to magnetically bind to toxins and pull them out of the body. Many spas have clay baths, clay body wraps, facial clay cleansers and masks. People have rubbed mud / clay on their bodies for centuries knowing it will make their skin look and feel amazing. Drinking clay in moderation is also healthy. Clay will bind to all the toxins and help pull them out of my body. I make sure to buy an edible brand. Although all clay is edible, I want to make sure the processing of the clay is natural.

HOW TO EAT: Mix 1 teaspoon of clay in water and drink. Tastes like chalky water. Tastes good and is easy to drink. Put clay on my body or on skin rashes, skin growths or tumors as a poultice to pull the toxins out through my skin. Put a few tablespoons into my bath and soak.

6. PSYLLIUM HUSK

Shredded psyllium seeds are fiber that help scrape my intestines and my entire digestive track. Wet psyllium becomes gelatinous and heals my digestive track. It bulks up inside my system, so is great in making me feel more full during my cleanse. It thickens up any liquid I add it to, so I need to make sure to drink my psyllium drink quickly or I will be eating it with a spoon.

HOW TO EAT: Mix 1 teaspoon into water, juice or a smoothie. Drink fast or it will thicken. Drink lots of water to follow so the psyllium can move through my system and do its work.

7. ALOE VERA GEL

Peel my own aloe leaf by taking off the green cover and revealing the slimy gel filet on the inside or buy aloe gel bottles at health food stores. Aloe is super powerful at healing my inflamed digestive track and taking the fire of my body down. It alkalines and soothes my body. I can blend it into smoothies or juices. It is flavorless but can be bitter and is amazing for my skin glow also.

HOW TO EAT: Buy as a juice and do shooters daily or break a leaf off my plant and filet it. Blend aloe in juice or any liquid and drink.

8. TURMERIC CURCUMIN

A root which grows much like ginger underground and is one of the most powerful healing plants of inflammation on the planet. It reduces inflammation in my body and studies have proven, curcumin can heal cancer. In order for the healing powers to be effective, it should be mixed with black pepper to release the medicine. I can buy as pills, in powder form or as a root in the produce section of the grocery store. From now on, I will add turmeric to EVERYTHING. I add the powder to my savory meals and into my sauces and dressings. I make Petra's tea recipe with the roots and add it to my juices and smoothies. It is very orange and stains everything. Curcumin is the active ingredient inside turmeric that has been proven to help cancer healing and greatly reduce inflammation in the body. Since inflammation is at the stem of most sickness, including cancer, it makes sense this medicine can help heal me.

HOW TO EAT: :   Buy pills with high concentration of curcumin including black pepper or take with black pepper for full medicine activation.   Sprinkle turmeric powder on my food.   Add the root to my smoothies, juices, salads and stir fry's. Grate the root along with ginger and boil in water to make Petra's amazing healing tea, recipe in upcoming chapters.

9. HEMP CBD OIL

I have cannabinoid receptors in my body that want this medicine to feel good. Hemp is a cousin to the marijuana plant but does not get me high. Edible hemp seeds come from this hemp plant. Hemp is also used to make clothing, rope, houses, shoes, cars and paper. It is the only plant that gives nutrients back to the soil and could help save our world. It could replace us pillaging our forests, momma earth and heal our lands back again. It was once a mandatory crop for all USA farmers but is now banned across the world as pharmaceutical companies and big lumber corporations know it would put them out of business.

Ingesting CBD oil instantly supports my neurological system, muscles and my brain into relaxation mode. It can help with PTSD, stress, trauma, anxiety, depression, seizures, insomnia, Alzheimer's, cancer, body pain, heart pain and life pain. I can find it online and in dispensary shops as over the counter medicine. It is safe for children, animals, older people and me. I promise that I will explore and try this new (actually ancient) way of healing myself.

HOW TO EAT: It comes in liquid tinctures to drop under my tongue, pill capsules and also a cartridges for vape pens. I find a reliable source with CBD that is available for my body to absorb. There are many brands yet only some will really make a miraculous difference in my body.

A LOVE NOTE FROM PETRA: Hemp is a miraculous plant and if everyone took CBD oil for a few months to a few years, people and our society would be healed. With the high stresses of the world and our lives, it is important to have a natural way to relax, feel good in our body and in our mind. CBD helps relax our body, our heart and our neurological system. I believe the hemp and marijuana plant have been put on this earth as a way to help our consciousness and our bodies be healthy. I also believe the governments, money hungry corporations and world powers to be know this and that is why they have kept it under lock and key. Be good to yourself, eat cbd and hemp, heal your beautiful body back to your super human state so you are thriving on this planet. You are worth it! Private message me on Facebook for reliable sources of CBD oil, as some are not very effective.

- - ♥ - -

10. CHLORELLA

An algae that comes from lakes that is super powerful in removing heavy metals out of my body. It is a natural chelator along with cilantro. I might like or not like the taste. It is quite strong on its own yet I might love chewing the chlorella tablets.

HOW TO EAT: Buy it as a powder or chewable little tablets. Mix the powder in water and squeeze in fresh lemon to make it taste better. It smells a little like dirty socks but makin it into a lemony drink tastes quite good. Some people love the taste and will munch on chlorella tablets by the handfuls all day.

A LOVE NOTE FROM PETRA: I drank mass amounts of chlorella lemon water when I had my amalgam mercury fillings removed, so I could get all the excess metals out of my body. I don't love the taste of the tablets, so I have become creative as I know the healing effects of this power plant. I stuff chlorophyll tablets into sundried olives which tastes quite yummy or I eat the tablets along with other food so I can't really taste them. I also drink chlorella lemon water which tastes good to me.

- - ♥ - -

11. SPIRULINA

A powerhouse green algae that studies state could be sold for $100 per pill based on the amount of healing it can do for the body. It is super high in protein. Ounce per ounce, 100 X more protein than steak. It is extremely alkaline for the body and a super source of chlorophyll. Vegan body builders consume high levels of spirulina to keep their protein levels up. It makes a great green drink mixed with lemon spring water and tastes cheezy added to salads, popcorn and other meals. Can also add it to smoothies to make them more green and nutrient packed.

HOW TO EAT: Buy it as a powder and make into green drinks with lemons and spring water. Add to green smoothies. Sprinkle on top of popcorn and salads. Add it where you can use an extra mineral and chlorophyll boost.

A LOVE NOTE FROM PETRA: I don't add spirulina to my green smoothies as I prefer them to taste yummy and spirulina does alter their taste. I prefer drinking it as a lemony drink or adding it to food. It does taste really good on popcorn with nutritional yeast (hippie cheese) as it tastes cheezy.

- - ♡ - -

12. WHEATGRASS

A grass I can grow and juice at home or buy shooters at the juice shops. Used in cancer healing centers to quickly alkaline the body and kick it into healing mode. It is a simple grass to grow and comes from wheat berries. I can grow on my kitchen counter or on shoe racks in my house. It is packed full of protein, mass amounts of chlorophyll and tons of minerals for my expedited cleansing and healing. It is packed full of protein so an amazing addition to my plant based lifestyle. Vegan athletes drink lots of wheatgrass to keep their protein levels up. It is one of the most powerful grasses (along with alfalfa) on the planet so will quickly take my cleansing / healing journey to the next level. The taste is quite intense and can make me nauseous if I am not used to this level of cleansing. If I feel sick after drinking it, it is not an indication that the wheatgrass is bad for me but that my body is not at this level of health yet. So I am gentle with myself, I can dilute the shot with water and also drink it after I've had a few juices or a little solid food.

HOW TO EAT: Grow my own wheatgrass trays and cut the grass just above the dirt level then juice it in a wheatgrass or greens juicer. I can buy shots in juice bars and I make sure to ask for them to be juiced fresh right in front of me. Some shops will have ready shots sitting in the fridge but fresh is where the medicine is, so I insist on this for my healing.

A LOVE NOTE FROM PETRA: Wheatgrass tastes really strong so I love drinking it like a tequila shot. My juicing clients love it this way too and it makes taking this medicine so much easier and more fun. We lick salt first on our hand, shoot the wheatgrass and then suck on a lime. We cheers our accomplishment. It's funny some people think it tastes delicious and others cringe. I don't love it, sometimes my body cringes and I get full body goose bumps yet I know the cleansing power so I go for it during my cleanses.

CHAPTER 22

SAMPLE CLEANSE DAYS

SAMPLE 1 - JUICY FOOD CLEANSE

This cleanse is the easiest because I get to eat solid raw food. If I am not ready to give up chewing, then this sample cleanse will be best for me. I am still giving my digestive system a break for most of the day, but adding in raw crunchy salads for a few meals. As long as I can keep it raw, I will expedite my healing. If I need to add cooked quinoa, potatoes, rice or veggies to my cleanse then it will help ease me into cleansing but slow down the healing process.

WAKE UP: and cleanse my mouth. Go poo with feet up on a pooping stool

DRINK: lemon water or apple cider vinegar water

CONNECT: to myself, meditate, ground into my body

COUNT: out loud 10 things I am grateful for

BREAKFAST: 1 glass green smoothie

10AM: 1 bowl JUICY chopped fruit

11AM: 1 glass fresh juice

12NN: 1 bowl big kickass salad with fresh homemade dressing

1PM: 1 cup hot tea elixir with nut mylk

2PM: 1 glass spring water or filtered water

3PM: Charcoal water or diatomaceous earth water

4PM: 1 glass fresh juice

5PM: 1 cup hot raw Soup

6PM: 1 bowl big kickass salad with fresh homemade dressing

7PM: 1 glass chocolate almond mylk

8PM: 1 bowl JUICY fresh fruit

9PM: Magnesium capsules to oxygenate the colon

JUICY FOOD CLEANSE TIPS...

- Eat as light and easy to digest food as possible in order to create a cleansing effect within my body even if I am eating solid food. Eat JUICY FOOD when eating solid food so I still get lots of hydration inside my body.

- Get creative with my blender and make liquid food as much as possible.

- Add cooked quinoa, rice, potatoes or veggies if I need the extra bulk. I let go of eating food as my cleanse transitions to create the highest healing effect and I let go of cooked food for my cleanse to expedite.

- Add a nap in throughout the day, take time to close my eyes even if I'm just sitting. Ideally go to sleep before 11pm.

- On Days 3 add in a colonic with a Colon Hydro Therapist

- On Days 2 and 5 add in coffee or water enema with myself

- Look in the mirror and tell myself, "I am proud of me. It takes courage to cleanse, to let go and to change something. I am brave and I can do this. I am totally worth it."

- Look in the mirror again and tell myself "I love myself radically and I practice in every moment to love myself more. I am great. I stretch my body. I breathe. I take really good care of myself. I take baths. I think happier thoughts. I release all negative un serving habits and beliefs. I am totally worth it."

SAMPLE 2 - JUICY LIQUID CLEANSE

In this cleanse I drink various liquids and don't eat any food. I can add in more fatty protein smoothies, nut mylks and green smoothies. In the blender I can make easy JUICY food that will cleanse me.

WAKE UP: and cleanse my mouth. Go poo with feet up on a pooping stool

DRINK: lemon water or apple cider vinegar water

CONNECT: to myself, meditate, ground into my body

COUNT: out loud 10 things I am grateful for

BREAKFAST: 1 glass green smoothie

10AM: Charcoal water or diatomaceous earth water

11AM: 1 glass fresh juice

12NN: 1 glass protein mylk fatty smoothie

1PM: 1 glass spring water or filtered water

2PM: 1 glass fresh juice

3PM: Charcoal water or diatomaceous earth water

4PM: 1 cup hot tea elixir

5PM: 1 glass spring water or filtered water

6PM: 1 glass savoury veggie green smoothie or hot raw soup

7PM: 1 cup fresh nut mylk

8PM: 1 glass spring water or filtered water

9PM: Magnesium capsules to oxygenate the colon

JUICY LIQUID CLEANSE TIPS...

- This is a great base LIQUID cleanse guideline. Add in or take out as I feel. Add more mylks, protein smoothies, raw soups or hot tea elixirs to ease into cleanse. Add in more juices, spring water and coconut water to expedite my healing.

- Get creative with making liquid food in the blender

- This cleanse will give my digestive system a break

- Add a nap in throughout the day, take time to close my eyes even if I'm just sitting. Ideally go to sleep before 11pm.

- On Days 3 and 5 add in a colonic with a Colon Hydro Therapist

- On Days 2 and 7 add in coffee enema with myself

- Add in more psyllium husk to water, juices or liquid drinks to create more bulk and sustenance so I am less hungry. It will help scrape my intestines.

- Look in the mirror and tell myself, "I am proud of me. It takes courage to cleanse, to let go and to change something. I am brave and I can do this. I am totally worth it."

- Look in the mirror again and tell myself "I love myself radically and I practice in every moment to love myself more. I am great. I stretch my body. I breathe. I take really good care of myself. I take baths. I think happier thoughts. I release all negative un serving habits and beliefs. I am totally worth it."

SAMPLE 3 – JUICY JUICE CLEANSE

This is one sample of a JUICY juice cleanse I can do that focuses on drinking juices and eating no food. I can add in more or take drinks out. I can also add a green smoothie in the mornings and a raw soup or protein smoothie in the evening. This is a guideline for me to create the perfect cleanse for myself based on all the information I learn from this book as my guide. I can do this! The more I want to cleanse, the more leave the fat and fibre out.

WAKE UP: and cleanse my mouth. Go poo with feet up on a pooping stool

DRINK: lemon water or apple cider vinegar water

CONNECT: to myself, meditate, ground into my body

COUNT: out loud 10 things I am grateful for

BREAKFAST: 1 glass fresh juice

10AM: Charcoal water or diatomaceous earth water

11AM: 1 glass spring water or filtered water

12NN: 1 glass fresh juice

1PM: 1 cup herbal tea (add nut mylk if I want more gentle)

2PM: 1 glass fresh juice

3PM: 1 glass spring water with charcoal or diatomaceous earth

4PM: 1 glass fresh juice

5PM: 1 glass spring water or filtered water

6PM: 1 glass psyllium husk water or juice

7PM: 1 cup herbal tea (add nut mylk if I want more gentle)

8PM: 1 glass fresh juice

9PM: Magnesium capsules to oxygenate the colon

JUICY JUICE CLEANSE TIPS...

- This is a great base juice cleanse guideline. Add in or take out as I feel. Add more fresh mylks and hot tea elixirs to ease myself into the cleanse or go green juice and water only to expedite my healing.

- Replace juice or water with coconut water as often as you want.

- Add a nap in throughout the day, take time to close my eyes even if I'm just sitting. Ideally go to sleep before 11pm.

- On Days 3, 5 and 7 add in a colonic with a Colon Hydro Therapist

- On Days 2, 4 and 6 add in a coffee enema with myself

- Add more psyllium husk to water, juices or liquid drinks to create more bulk and sustenance so I am less hungry. It will help scrape my intestines.

- Look in the mirror and tell myself, "I am proud of me. It takes courage to cleanse, to let go and to change something. I am brave and I can do this. I am totally worth it."

- Look in the mirror again and tell myself "I love myself radically and I practice in every moment to love myself more. I am great. I stretch my body. I breathe. I take really good care of myself. I take baths. I think happier thoughts. I release all negative un serving habits and beliefs. I am totally worth it."

CHAPTER 23

MORE JUICY TIPS FOR SUCCESS

- Cleansing is not starving. I fill myself up with JUICY liquids that are full of nutrition. I cannot starve drinking so many super liquids.

- Fill in my day with more juices and more smoothies as I feel I need to stay full and satiated.

- Drink lots of water and lots of water in between my juices.

- Drink fresh coconut water in between my juices or do a coconut water only cleanse.

- Drink MORE vegetable and green juices.

- Drink LESS fruit juices. Fruit juices will spike my sugar levels, crash me and not give me as much nutrition to sustain me.

- Avoid pasteurized juices which are acidic to my body.

- Cut out soda pop, bottled fruit juice, coffee, black tea, alcohol and processed sugary drinks that are acidic to my body and will harm me instead of doing me good.

- Avoid wheat, dairy, soy, sugar, coffee, alcohol, processed food and meat to create a cleansing experience for my body.

- Add other kinds of liquids into my cleanse as long as they are healthy, alkaline and fresh.

- If I need to satiate myself more, I add almond or coconut mylk, teas, fatty elixirs, raw soups, veggie broths and any other liquids that will cleanse, hydrate and alkaline me.

- Good fats will help fill me up like avocado, coconut yogurt, almond mylk, coconut mylk, coconut oil and hemp seeds. Each of these can be added to my smoothies or liquid drink creations.

- Nut mylks and fatty smoothies will fill me up more.

- Cut up juicy fruit for snacking and store in fridge.

- If I am eating a little during my cleanse, then I eat smaller easy to digest meals if I feel hungry so my body still gets a break from digesting.

- Quinoa is an alkaline grain, easy to digest and fills me up. Make a pot of this and have in fridge if I need food to snack on. Heat and eat with Himalayan salt and little bit olive oil. If salads are part of my JUICY cleanse, then I can add quinoa on top of my salad.

- Blend frozen bananas in blender with a few spoons of water for a light snack as this will make banana ice cream. Add additional frozen fruit and I have sorbet. Add raw cacao or chia seeds or shredded coconut for extra yum. This is a great easy to make dessert that is very JUICY. More ice cream recipes in upcoming chapters.

- Eat chopped veggies with natural hummus (no canola oil) for my hunger pangs if I am incorporating food.

- Cut avocado in ½ , add salt and lemon juice to make a great fatty healthy snack.

- Rest as much as possible to love on my body. My energy might drop before it increases. I am gentle with myself. I love on myself. I take care of myself. I nurture myself.

- I don't have to drink just juices to be cleansing. I can cut out a few harmful items for a week or two and I am rocking a cleanse. Easy breezy! Take my health into my hands and do this, I am WORTH it! My body LOVES me.

- Put a jug of water into the fridge for making cold smoothies every morning.

- Let my bananas brown with few spots, peel them and place in ziploc bag into the freezer for smoothie ingredients.

- Buy frozen fruit to have as back up to store in my freezer. Frozen mangos, pineapples, strawberries, peaches and blueberries are best for smoothie making.

- Slice up my lemons for the week, for morning lemon water.

- Make a pot herbal delicious tea, add lemon and a sweetener and store in fridge for a cold drink.

- Freeze my green smoothies if time is an issue. Make a container of green smoothie and place in ziploc freezer bags into the freezer. That way if I am in a rush, I can pull a bag out the night prior or first thing in the morning to defrost. Fresh is always best but sometimes I need time and convenience on my side.

- Stock up my fridge full of veggies and fruit. Prep and chop up what I need. It is easy to stay on the healthy path when I open my fridge and have stuff to grab.

- Allocate time in the morning to make all my juices for the day or for part of the day. Have several juices in the fridge so I always have something to grab.

- Make nut mylks or teas and store in the fridge to have more liquid options.

- Set my intentions, commit to cleansing and fill in my intention questions. Once I choose to do it, then I do it.

- Find a buddy to cleanse with, ideally in the same house or a coworker. It makes it easier to have someone for moral support and to also alternate the juice making process. It is fun to make juices for my buddy one day and they make juices for me the next day. And I can totally do this on my own. I am that powerful!

CHAPTER 24

JUICE DELIVERY

F OR MY JUICY CLEANSE, I CAN MAKE MY OWN juices or have them delivered from a juice shop. The most convenient option is to have juices delivered to me. It will ensure my fastest success and keep me better on track. If I can afford a juice delivery, then I start with this option to try JUICY cleansing for the first time. I will have 5 juices delivered to me daily. It will ensure I am well fed and on track for my cleansing regime.

However, ordering juices can be expensive and making my own is more cost effective if I am not accounting for my own time spent making the juices. Making my own juices is simple, so I don't get scared to do it on my own. I will need to do daily preparation and planning to ensure my cleansing success.

I can also have some combination of delivery and make my own to make my life simpler. How I want to set up my JUICY cleansing week is up to me. But most important, I set it up and I do it. My health is waiting for me to take it to the next level. So I make it happen.

Research juice delivery places in my area for the convenience of ordering juices to my house. Having juices delivered daily or for the first 1 or 2 days of my cleanse will be really helpful. Some juice shops are set up for pick up only so every morning I would go pick up my fresh juices for the day. Also research juice shops or grocery stores that make fresh juices. That way if I am making my own and buying some, I can plan out my excursions to include a fresh juice shop. Maybe I make a morning juice and buy a juice for lunch and then get home to make my dinner juice. This juicing plan is up to me so I strategize and get myself organized so I ensure my success. If I know where to buy my juices, I won't go hungry and I won't cheat. The worst punisher is my own guilt when I start out planning to do a JUICY cleanse, but then due to starvation or lack of convenience, I stray. I love myself enough to set myself up and organize my juices ahead of time.

TIPS FOR JUICE DELIVERY...

TIP #1:
Don't have juices delivered for more than 2 days at a time. Most delivery places want to make the juices and deliver me 5 days worth, which saves them time but I WANT LIFEFORCE and old juices no longer have it. So I insist on fresh and get no more than 2 days for delivery. If I can pick up or have juices delivered daily, this is my best option for life force, healing power juice.

TIP #2:

Find places around town that sell fresh juices and smoothies. This will make it easier for me when I am on the go but want to Eat Juicy! Most organic health grocery stores have fresh smoothies and fresh juices for sale. Natural Markets and many other grocery stores make them.

TIP #3:

Buy a wheat grass shot every day or every other day while I am on this JUICY cleanse. This super strong alkaline green drink will do wonders for my body. It is one of the most potent greens on the planet and will give me even more healing than green juices and green smoothies. The taste is strong, I can chase it with an orange slice, lemon or fresh juice. I might cringe, get goose bumps but it's worth it. Cancer healing centers all over the world offer this powerful drink as part of the daily cleansing and healing regime.

TIP #4:

Even the not so healthy smoothie places like Jamba Juice (in USA), now have kale smoothies. They may not be organic but they do the trick. I ask for fresh kale/greens to be added as some use a frozen mix. To keep my juice healthy and alkaline, ask for coconut water or water as my base instead of the acidic pasteurized bottled fruit juice they use. Look for juice and smoothie shops popping up at airports, food courts and around town. I always ask for the list of ingredients and ask how they will make my beverage. Then adjust the recipe to make it healthier.

TIP #5:

Stay away from cold press juices if I can buy freshly squeezed juices instead. Most of the life force is missing in cold press juices as they usually sit for many hours on the shelf. Most cold press juice shops make their juice the night prior, so when I buy it in the morning it is already 12 or more hours old. The store will state that the nutrients are still in tact, but I can taste the OLD of the juice. So if they have juices on a shelf, ask them to make me a fresh one instead. Same with wheatgrass shots, I always ask for fresh.

TIP #6:

Juices lose their vitamin and life force content within minutes of being juiced. So I drink my juices fresh and drink them right away. When I finish making my juice, I drink it first and then clean my juicer. I get the life force inside of me as fast as possible. If I am making juice for a juice cleanse, then I will need to make a couple of jars at the same time for my convenience and to take juice with me to work. I will likely make all my juices in the morning so I can save time throughout the day. Then I can order juices to fill my day's JUICY menu. Prepping myself and grocery shopping ahead of time, will really help me be successful.

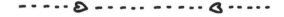

CHAPTER 25

GROCERY SHOPPING

THIS CHAPTER IS A SHOPPING GUIDELINE for me depending on what veggies and fruits I like, what kinds of juices or smoothies I plan to make, the level of cleanse I am choosing and how much I plan to consume.

I will need to do daily preparation and planning to ensure my cleansing success.

This is a rough guideline of items to buy instead of a direct shopping list, as the amounts and ingredients will be up to me and my plan for my cleansing week.

If I plan to do lots of juicing, I will need lots of produce. If I plan to buy some juices or have them delivered, I will need less produce. Also if I plan to make smoothies, they require less produce than juices.

Perhaps I do my first shop and see how I go with the goods I purchased, then I can buy more as I need.

This is EXCITING!!!!!   I am GOING to buy yummy fruits and vegetables to fill up my fridge.

A bunch of JUICY food that will hydrate and nourish my BODY and SOUL! Yipeeee!!!

Ok let's GO SHOPPING!!!

HOW TO READ LABELS

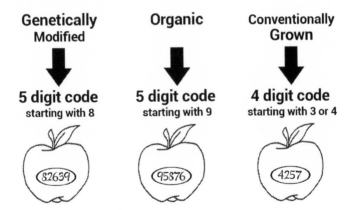

Genetically Modified	**Organic**	**Conventionally** Grown
5 digit code starting with 8	**5 digit code** starting with 9	**4 digit code** starting with 3 or 4
82639	95876	4257

PLACES TO SHOP...

(In order of preference):

1. MY OWN GARDEN – If I can grow fruits and vegetables in my back yard or grow sprouts and wheatgrass in my apartment, then I have the BEST GROCERY STORE EVER. I might not have time to grow a garden before my cleanse, yet I can plant for my future garden now. If I have friends with gardens, then I go raid theirs. Food picked and eaten fresh has the most amount of life force energy, digestive enzymes and vitamins.

2. FARMERS MARKETS – Find out when and where the farmers markets are in my area. Go shop there! The produce is the FRESHEST and has the most amount of life force as it was likely picked that morning. Plus I am supporting local farming, small businesses and people rather than corporations. This is also the best form of shopping therapy, bringing home bags and bags of fresh earth grown goodies. Buy organic or non sprayed if my budget can allow. Some fruit may not be certified organic but is tree ripened and only sprayed at blossom, this is better than conventional. The longer fruit can ripen on a tree, the healthier it is for my body to consume. Avoid buying fruit and vegetables that were picked green and ripened during the drive across the country in a truck. Some fruit and vegetables are also radiated when crossing borders, so it is best to buy local as much as possible.

3. FOOD COOPS & NATURAL GROCERY STORES Food coops are stores that are usually owned by the community or have the community on the board to make decisions. Most coops or natural grocers have a small store feel and usually care more about the well being of me as a customer. Their focus is to have healthy, organic, locally sourced and ethical products in their stores. They sell lots of organic, gluten free, dairy free and chemical free options. I always read ingredients of everything I buy. Just because it is sold in a healthier grocery store, doesn't mean it has the healthiest ingredients. I avoid canola oil, white sugar, white salt, white flour and preservatives still sneaking their way in to the healthier brands.

A LOVE NOTE FROM PETRA: I am very happy and pleasantly surprised that there are more and more of the healthier, natural, more conscious grocery stores around the world. I hold the intention that these kinder and more conscious health stores take over the world and people are no longer brainwashed to eat the chemical food that they thought was their only option. I hold the intention that we all awaken to what is real food that can heal us and what is fake food that is killing us....and stop buying that crap!

- - ♡ - -

4. CONVENTIONAL GROCERY STORES - Many conventional grocery stores are adding organic and natural food sections. Yipeee!!! Even Costco and big bulk stores stock much more healthy food. Yipeee!!! Conventional grocery stores should be last on my shopping list because most of their produce is not that fresh. It is picked prematurely and ripens on trucks and ships being transported across the country. If produce comes from USA and is heading into Canada for example, it is radiated (microwaved) before it can cross the border. Food in these stores has less life force and could be loaded with radiation energy. Of course, I do the best I can do. If conventional grocery stores are my only option and wilted kale is all I can get, then I rock it anyway. I still become healthier and cleanse my body by feeding it veggies, greens and fruit so I don't let the type of grocery store get in my way. I do what I can with what I have and I GO FOR IT!!! I read ingredients of all the products I buy, and especially important in these conventional grocery stores as they allow much more toxic chemical food to be sold. These stores are great however for buying frozen fruit for my fruit smoothies. Most of the time, they sell organic too. Costco (USA & Canada) sells big bags of frozen organic fruit for great prices. This makes my green smoothie lifestyle cost effective and convenient.

BUY THIS FOR MY JUICY CLEANSE...

1. LOTS OF LEAFY GREENS – Buy bunches of kale, spinach, cilantro, collards, romaine lettuce, bok choy, mint, parsley, wheatgrass, etc. Green leaves are packed with chlorophyll, which will naturally clean my blood, alkaline my body, boost my immune system and cleanse my body the fastest. Chlorophyll which is the blood of the leaf, is 99.9% the same as my human blood (hemoglobin). Chlorophyll and hemoglobin are composed of the same four elements – carbon, hydrogen, oxygen and nitrogen. The .1% difference is that hemoglobin is built around iron and chlorophyll is built around magnesium. They are almost the same liquid. So when I drink a green juice, it goes directly into my blood stream and cleans my blood. Drinking a green juice is a natural blood transfusion and the best cleanser for my body.

2. LOTS OF FRUIT – Ripe bananas and all other variety of fruit: pineapple, apples, lemons, limes, berries, mangos, watermelon, grapes, oranges, mandarins, whole coconuts, etc. Use fruit to sweeten the taste of my veggie juices and green smoothies, but I avoid cleansing on just fruit. Although many people feel great cleansing on just fruit, it spikes my glycemic levels and puts too much sugar into my system. Best to use the fruit as a snack or in combination with veggies and leaves to balance my blood sugar levels.

   If I choose to snack on fruit, then choose fruit that is super juicy and I can use my mouth as my juicer. Chew, chew, chew so I am swallowing juice rather than big un chewed chunks from eating too fast. Fruit is sugar. Although a healthier sugar than the processed white kind, it is still sugar. When I eat fruit whole or in smoothies, the fiber helps me balance out the sugar levels. When I juice fruit and remove the fibre, the juice will spike my glycemic levels quickly. Although I am juicing and doing something healthy for my body, too much sugar is not good for my body and will eventually cause me harm. I am aware to eat and drink in balance and love myself at the same time.

A LOVE NOTE FROM PETRA: I don't believe in the fruitarian diet, where they eat mostly boxes and boxes of fruit only. Eventually, I think this level of fructose in the body will create deterioration. I can eat a whole watermelon and feel great. If I juice the watermelon, it concentrates the sugars and I feel nauseous from this level of fructose in my body. Dried fruit is the same as all the water is dehydrated out of the fruit making the sugar levels extremely concentrated. So snacking too much on dried fruit is like eating candy and although it is healthier than candy, our body does not need excess sugar for thriving. Our body needs chlorophyll and good sources of fat. That is the ultimate diet in my opinion and the one I, personally, feel the best on. I eat fruit too and prefer the juicy watery fruits the best!

- - ♥ - -

3. LOTS OF VEGGIES – Celery, cucumber, beets, carrots, zucchini, avocado, tomatoes, cabbage, jicama, etc. Perfect for making veggie juices, kick ass salads and munching snacks. Most veggies are full of water and great for juicing. Veggies are nature's medicine along with leafy greens. Ideally veggies and greens are the biggest ingredients in my JUICY cleanse and in my JUICY lifestyle moving forward. If I plan to eat salads during my cleanse, then I prep, grate and chop my veggies into containers and store in my fridge. It will make my life and cleanse so much easier to have food ready and on hand when I feel snackish or ready to make juice. This will ensure success for me as well and keep me from getting hungry.

    I can grate or spirulize my beets, carrots, zucchini and jicama ahead of time and store in containers. They are easier to digest in this way and much more fun to eat. If I have not tried jicama then I go get some right now. It looks like a white turnip and is sold in most grocery stores and Asian markets. I might have seen it but never thought about buying it. The skin peels of simple with a knife. It tastes like a cross between a crunchy apple and juicy edible potato. It is crunchy and super juicy. It is awesome for salads and dips and can also be cooked like a potato, but best eaten raw. It might become my favorite veggie to eat. Also celery has a strong taste and can alter the taste of my juices too much. I try juicing celery on its own for an extra healing drink and great body mineral boost.

4. LOTS OF GREEN APPLES – Apples go perfect with green leaves and veggies to sweeten up my juices without

adding too much sugar content. They are slightly sweet and sour at the same time, making my juices even yummier. If I plan to eat solid food during my cleanse or want a great munching snack for my future JUICY lifestyle, then I slice apples and dip them into almond butter and then coat them with hemp seeds, shredded coconut, raw cacao or any other yummy super food.

5. LOTS OF ORANGES, PINEAPPLES, CITRUS – I use oranges, apples, pineapples and grapefruits to sweeten up my green juices and make them easier and more fun to drink. They are also great if I get hungry during my cleanse and want a little solid JUICY food to munch on. Pomelos are another great JUICY fruit for satiation and fun. They are like a very giant grapefruit but much sweeter with a firmer texture I can bite into. If I am cutting sugar out completely during my cleanse, then I use lemons instead to reduce the green taste of my juices.

6. LOTS OF CUCUMBERS – For juices, salads and JUICY snacking, as they are full of liquid and are a great way to add hydration to my body. Cucumbers are great for the skin and soothing my digestive track. They don't require much digesting power so I snack on them. I can also add cucumbers to my juices to create larger quantities as they are so full of water. An easy snack is sliced cucumbers sprinkled with pink Himalayan salt and pepper.

7. LOTS OF CARROTS – For juices and shredded in salads. They are also amazing for my body and straight carrot juice is delicious and extremely healing for me. Combine them with apples or oranges and ginger for the yummiest juice

ever. Also use carrots to help move my other produce through the juicer. Because they are hard, a few pieces added in throughout juicing other veggies and green leaves, helps push the produce through the juicer to ensure nothing gets stuck. If I have experience in juicing, then I know that having to stop in the middle of my juicing process to unclog and clean the juicer is a pain. So I juice slowly and use carrots to keep the juicer clean and everything moving. Straight carrot juice has been used for cancer healing. Carrots are root vegetables and will convert to sugar in the body, yet the power of these sugars seem to be fighting cancer rather than feeding it.

8. LOTS OF LEMONS & LIMES – For juices, smoothies and lemon water in the morning. Lemons are the most alkaline fruit on the planet, along with watermelons. They are acidic by nature but once they touch my lips, they turn alkaline. Making lemon water first thing in the morning will be my new best friend. Lemons are amazing for juices as they cut the green taste and make my juice and smoothies taste much more delicious. They are a staple for my cleanse and new JUICY lifestyle forever and ever.

9. LOTS OF GINGER & TURMERIC ROOT – For juices, smoothies and making healing teas. Ginger and turmeric are super powerful medicines. Ginger is very good for the digestive system and for my body overall. Turmeric is anti inflammatory and cancer healing. Add a few nubs to juices and smoothies depending on how spicy I want it as ginger is spicy. Grate a few nubs and boil in water to make Petra's most healing tea (recipe in upcoming chapters).

CHAPTER 26

BUY ORGANIC VS CONVENTIONAL

F I CAN AFFORD TO BUY ORGANIC then I always choose this option. Most conventional vegetables are heavily sprayed and have tons of left over pesticides on the skin, which may penetrate into the fruit.

If I can't afford all organic, then conventional produce is ok too especially for juicing as I am tossing out the pulp and skins. When I juice I need a lot of ingredients, so buying a combination of organic and conventional can make it more affordable for me. It is safer to buy conventional produce with peels like oranges, lemons, grapefruits, watermelon and bananas as I will peel them. Ideally all my leafy greens, apples and vegetables I buy organic. Conventional produce is grown in chemical, not very nutritious soil, so it is not the best choice for my JUICY lifestyle. The ideal scenario is that the toxins have not gotten inside the fruit or nature has a way of filtering them out. Buying lots of produce can be expensive, so I do the best I can. I am still doing more good for my body giving it vegetable juice than anything else, so I don't get hung up on organic vs. non organic. I buy what I can organic and bless the rest to be healthy for my body.

Most importantly, I remove toxic processed food out of my kitchen and start reading the ingredients of all my food before I buy it. I remove food like: white sugar, white flour, canola oil, high fructose corn syrup, MSG, aspartame, conventional corn and soy products (genetically modified), food colorings, artificial flavors and names I can't pronounce or understand. Food is my medicine so I use it to heal my body. The following foods are the ones I will buy organic when ever possible:

Buy This Organic
FOODS WITH THE MOST PESTICIDE RESIDUE

Strawberries
Apples
Celery
Sweet Bell Peppers
Peaches
Nectarines
Grapes
Spinach

CHAPTER 27

LET'S GET ME ORGANIZED

I N ORDER FOR ME TO BE SUCCESSFUL with my JUICY cleanse, I need to get organized. I either order juices ahead of time or I go buy all my ingredients. I spend time prepping and organizing my ingredients for my morning juicing or smoothie making routine.

As I continue into my new JUICY lifestyle, I will spend time weekly prepping my healthy ingredients and storing them in containers in the fridge. This simple act will increase my success of eating healthy as well as create convenience for my lifestyle. Every athlete who trains and eats with awareness, preps their meals to make their success more achievable. I will learn from them. Maybe I prep my veggies on the weekend to get ready for my upcoming work week or I prep when I get home from the grocery store. Prepping my fresh produce before putting it in the fridge might be easier for me. I can also make a big pot of soup, veggie stew or quinoa and portion it out for my daily lunches. By bringing healthy food with me to work, I will ensure I keep a JUICY HEALTHY VIBRANT lifestyle going. When I make my body my focus and recognize it as this incredible super computer spaceship temple that I (my soul) reside in, then I will feed it only the BEST food possible. I now make feeding myself nourishing food my priority!

During my JUICY cleanse, if I am making my own juices and smoothies, then I make sure my fridge is stocked. I don't need to cut or grate my produce in advance, I just give myself extra time to wash and chop my produce in the morning as I make my juice.

The easiest way to START is to fill a big bowl of produce for each flavor of juice I plan to make and line them up beside my juicer. I keep my red juices separate from my green juices, to create variety of colors to feed my eyes and a variety of flavors to feed my mouth and tummy. I create bright green, bright red and bright orange juices, instead of mixing everything together to make brown muddy juice. I first eat with my eyes, so my juices have to look appealing for me to get excited about drinking them. So first thing in the morning before juicing, I prep a big bowl of produce for my RED juice, a big bowl of produce for my ORANGE juice and a big bowl of produce for my GREEN juice.

GREEN JUICE BOWL: For Example.... chopped up kale, spinach, cilantro, parsley, cucumber, celery, green apple, ginger, lemons, limes

ORANGE JUICE BOWL: For Example... chopped up carrots, oranges, ginger, turmeric, fennel, lemons, limes

RED JUICE BOWL: For Example... chopped up beets, grapefruit, cabbage, watermelon, ginger, lemons, limes

I change the ingredients to adjust to my preferences. Chopping carrots and feeding them in to my juicer between my greens can be helpful in pushing the leaves through the juicer, preventing it from getting clogged. This will also depend on the type of juicer I have and how well it juices leaves.

MORE PREPPING TIPS...

JUICING

- Easiest to get my fruit and veggies ready right before I make my juice.

- Fill a sink full of water, wash all my ingredients, chop them and transfer to a bowl ready for juicing.

- Create a big bowl of one juice flavor / color ready for juicing.

- To keep my juice colors clean, I make my green juice first. I then run a little water through the juicer to clean it. I make my orange juice next. Run a little more water through. I make the red juice last as it's colors are the strongest and will affect all my other juices.

GREENS

- Keep dry so they don't rot.

- Wrap in paper towel or tea towel to pull moisture out.

- Store in sealed big plastic or glass containers.

- Store in plastic bag air tight once wrapped in tea towel.

- More details on storing greens in upcoming chapter.

VEGGIES

- Chop and prep my veggies to rock out salad making and to have healthy snacking food on hand.

- Buy hummus and other healthy dips for easy veggie snacks. Read the ingredients and avoid brands with canola oil and preservatives.

- Chop or grate carrots, beets, cabbage, cauliflower, broccoli, celery, cucumbers, peppers so they are ready for munching and instant meals.

- Prepping veggies is the most important part of maintaining my JUICY lifestyle. When I get home from work hungry, I won't feel like grating beets or chopping stuff up to make a salad. It is easier to have my storage containers in the fridge ready to make a quick salad, veggie wrap, stir fry or soup. I will ensure keeping my healthy lifestyle.

FRUIT

- Not all fruit works for prepping as it oxidizes easily.

- I can chop and prep: grapes, pineapple, oranges, watermelon and melons.

- Store in containers in my fridge so I always have snacks on hand.

SMOOTHIES

- Don't freeze greens as I am eating them for the life force value. Freezing greens devalues their nutritional content but sometimes convenience is helpful so instead of freezing greens, I freeze a ready made smoothie instead.

- Get greens as fresh as possible, ideally picked from a garden that morning or a few days prior. The fresher the greens, the more life force they have.

- Going on a road trip, camping or know I will not have a blender, then I make my smoothies ahead of time, pour them into Ziploc bags and freeze them. They will last well in a cooler and ensure healthy food on my travels.

- It's also convenient to chop and freeze my fruit for smoothies so they are always ready to go. Buy already brown bananas, peel and freeze them so I always have ingredients on hand. I will have to ask the grocer if they have any stored in the back as they only put out the very green or yellow bananas. The moment that the bananas start to ripen, they remove them to the back to be tossed out. Usually I can get a discount on brown or very yellow bananas.

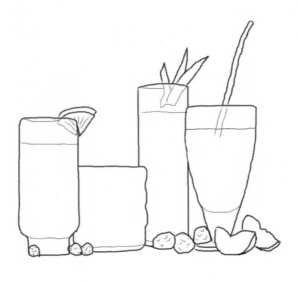

- - ♡ - -

CHAPTER 28

STORING
MY GREENS

I T SUCKS SPENDING MONEY ON ORGANIC KALE and spinach and having it go bad within a few days in the fridge. So using storing techniques for my greens, to make them last longer is essential in maintaining my JUICY lifestyle program.

One note about greens is, I always eat them as fresh as possible. Frozen spinach does not have the same life force like fresh and I want to eat as much life force as possible. The more life force energy I eat, the more alive and energized I will feel. Ideally I buy my greens at farmer's markets, so they are super fresh.

Sometimes I do what I can, in the busy lifestyle that I have to make healthy choices. If for convenience, I buy my greens in bulk grocery stores or non organic shops, that is ok.

I will attempt to find the organic greens or farm fresh greens next time. Most bagged greens are sprayed with a preservative to maintain their freshness and it is not ideal to ingest. So I buy bagged greens when I need to and I always choose farm fresh alternatives when I can.

With any greens I buy, I want to maintain their crispness and green chlorophyll color as long as possible. These 2 methods will ensure my greens are dry and protected from air, which will deteriorate them much faster.

STORING GREENS OPTION A...

1. Spread out my greens on a tea towel
2. Roll the tea towel up like a burrito enveloping my greens
3. Place burrito inside plastic bag and wrap it around to be air tight
4. Place in fridge

STORING GREENS OPTION B...

1. Spread one layer of greens inside a large plastic or glass storage container
2. Place a layer of paper towels on top of my greens
3. Spread second layer of greens on top of my paper towels
4. Place a layer of paper towels, continue alternating
5. Close container with airtight lid
6. Place in fridge

CHAPTER 29

KITCHEN EQUIPMENT

WHAT KIND OF JUICER SHOULD I BUY? The type of juicer can be important and yet I can get started with a simple $50 juicer. If I am willing to spend a few hundred dollars, I will get a much higher quality juicer. The difference between the cheaper juicer and more expensive one, will be how much juice it actually extracts from the produce and how much juice is still left in the pulp that I throw away. Basically the amount of juice yield and the dryness of my pulp. If the juicer is cheaper it will spin faster and not extract as much juice.

If juice is not extracted properly, my pulp will be wet and still full of juice. I can put my pulp back in through the juicer a few times to get more juice out. The slower more expensive juicers, create a very dry pulp and yield much more juice.

THERE ARE 3 KINDS OF JUICERS WITH 3 KINDS OF BLADES...

1. SHARP TEETH MESH STRAINER – price range $. This juicer rips the produce quickly with its sharp teeth. If I want fast juice with easy clean up, then I get this juicer. These juicers with teeth are much faster, but will heat my juice from the speed and also leave a lot of the liquid inside the pulp. My pulp will be more wet. Ideally I put the pulp back in through again to squeeze out the extra juice. The sharp teeth do not like celery as it is stringy and will tangle in the teeth of the blade, so I cut my celery very small. The teeth will not like greens either, so I chop them small too as the fibers of the greens can get tangled in the teeth also. I might need to strain the juice with a strainer to get out excess pulp that can sneak into the juice.

2. ONE GEAR – price range $$. Usually considered a cold press juicer. Moves much slower and extracts more juice out of the pulp. Pulp is pretty dry. Can be a little more complicated to clean with more pieces. Might still have to strain juice to get out excess pulp. Juices slower so does not heat up juice and makes more love to the produce so the result is perhaps a tastier juice. I will need to chop my produce and greens so they don't get tangled in the blade. I use chopped carrots to push my greens through to prevent my juicer from getting clogged. Some one gear juicers have an extra attachment blade I can purchase to make soft serve ice cream from frozen fruit. This is a great reason to choose this juicer.

HUROM OR KUVINGS JUICERS

These vertical juicers have a one gear wide blade that slowly presses my juice, leaving my pulp fairly dry. They are semi great for greens and other veggies. I always pour my finished juice through a strainer with these models, as they don't separate the pulp so well. Pouring through an extra strainer before drinking my juice, ensures I remove the pulp. There is nothing wrong with pulp, but I might not like floating chunky bits in my juices. I drink the pulp in my smoothies instead. The Kuvings model has an ice cream adapter I can buy. I can press frozen fruit through it to make sorbet. This is of course an incredible easy snack for my upcoming JUICY lifestyle.

3. TWO GEAR – price range $$. Much slower press. Extracts all juice out. Pulp is extra dry. Does greens the best. Can put in bigger pieces of vegetables and it handles it. Not great at doing tons of carrots as it moves so slow. Much better for greens. Can put in whole stalks of celery and wheatgrass. Simple daily juicer. Makes really tasty green juice.

OMEGA OR GREEN STAR JUICERS

These horizontal juicers with 2 gear blades are great for juicing greens. These super slow juicers don't heat my juice and really take time to wring out every drop of liquid, leaving my pulp waste very dry. Th two gears press the produce between them, instead of teeth that shred it.

OTHER EQUIPMENT...

NUTMYLK BAG

Total must have and must have several! Good to have 2 bags, one for pressing green juices and one for pressing nut mylks. This mesh strainer bag will help me stay on my healthy path. It's like a cheese cloth that I pour juices or nut mylks through to strain them. I squeeze the bag, milk my liquid and throw out the pulp. I can buy nutmylk bags at organic grocery stores or on amazon. I can make a green juice using my blender, by blending leafy greens, lemon and water. It turns into a not so pretty pulpy smoothie, I then pour it through my nut mylk bag. It separates the pulp from the liquid and I am left with a super quick and easy green juice without needing a juicer.

COCONUT OPENER

Makes life easier. Coconuts can be a part of my JUICY cleanse and lifestyle no matter where I am in the world. When buying my coconuts fresh in tropical places, they will open or partly open them for me for easy access. When on the mainland, I can buy coconuts at the Asian markets that are the Thai Coconuts wrapped in plastic wrap. Having the Coconut Jack to open these will make my world super easy. I can use a giant knife or a machete to hack my coconuts open on my kitchen countertop every morning, yet it might be a bit dangerous. So I will look into buying the cocojack. www.Coco-Jack.com

GRATER

Important to have, to grate ginger, turmeric and all kinds of veggies. A tool I will use all the time. I can buy larger ones for beets and carrots and smaller ones for ginger and lemon peel. A must have in my kitchen.

CITRUS JUICER

If I am making lots of citrus juice, I get an electric citrus juicer which is inexpensive to buy. For squeezing a few lemons or oranges, I buy a manual citrus press or corkscrew style tool that helps me get all the juice out.

A LOVE NOTE FROM PETRA: When I lived on Maui, I had an orchard full of oranges, lemons and pomelos, so having an electric juicer was awesome. I also use the wooden cork screw style tool for making my lemon water every morning. If I don't have any tools around, then using a spoon to squeeze out a lemon or orange is just as helpful.

- - ♡ - -

CERAMIC KNIFE

Sharp kitchen knives are the best. Dull knives in my kitchen are actually more dangerous than sharp ones. Dull knives don't grip and can easily slip on me. I sharpen all my kitchen metal knives and I buy a ceramic knife too. A ceramic knife is very sharp and I will love it, if I have not tried it yet. When my fruit and veggies never touch metal, there is less oxidization for the produce and it feels good to chop food with it. I am careful storing it as it is made of glass. Ceramic knives can chip and break very easily so I am more cautious. Some ceramic knives come with their own holder, making it easy to take my knife with me where ever I need.

VITAMIX HIGH SPEED BLENDER

A must have for my JUICY lifestyle. A high speed blender, makes food making super easy. It can hold more liquid than the average blender and blends everything super smooth. It can heat up to make hot raw drinks and is also strong enough to puree frozen fruit or ice to make ice cream. I will love this machine, if I don't already. Vitamix offers no interest payment plans or has refurbished models that were used in demos with 5 year warranties at discounted prices. They give a brand new pitcher so I would never know someone used it for a demo. I can go online or call their 1-800 number. www.Vitamix.com

BLENDTEC HIGH SPEED BLENDER

I will love this machine too. I either am a vitamix or a blendtec fan and this depends on my preference. Blendtec has preset buttons for convenience and is just as powerful. Call them for discounted models. www.Blendtec.com

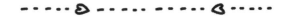

CHAPTER 30

SUPER FOODS

OODS TO ADD TO MY JUICY CLEANSE AND lifestyle. Super Foods are perfect for my new upcoming JUICY lifestyle, if I add them to my 7 + day JUICY cleanse is up to me. I can buy them all at healthier version grocery stores, some conventional supermarkets and online. I can use super foods as part of my cleanse or just add them to my JUICY lifestyle.

CHIA SEEDS

I will LOVE these little guys. Full of good oil and protein that gives me long lasting energy. Chia seeds become gelatinous when mixed with water. They help soothe my digestive track and bulk up my liquids. They are great to add to smoothies, desserts and to make chia pudding. Add to sweet stuff, cereals and smoothies. Thickens when wet and makes awesome VEGAN PROTEIN PACKED pudding.

HEMP SEEDS

Top SUPER FOOD! GET EM!!! Full of good oils, awesome source of plant based protein and CBD food that my body craves. Hemp seeds come from the hemp plant which is one of the most miraculous plants on the planet. Hemp can make clothes, rope, paper, shoes, houses and is one of the only plants that give nutrients back into the soil.

I can put hemp seeds on almost all my food to add protein, nutrition and good oils to my dishes and smoothies. I can blend 2 teaspoons with water in a blender and have instant hemp nut mylk. No straining needed.

Add hemp seeds to salads, pasta, pizza, sandwiches, wraps, smoothies, hot tea elixirs and anywhere I want to add extra nutrition. Make super easy quick hemp mylk.

APPLE CIDER VINEGAR

Add a capful into a glass of spring water for an amazing alkaline drink. Make sure I get raw apple cider vinegar, with the "mother" floating inside.

A favorite brand of many is called Braggs. I can drink a glass of apple cider water in the mornings or throughout the day to help alkaline my body and heal my digestive track. It is the best vinegar for salad dressings as it is alkaline and healing to eat.

RAW CACAO

Raw CHOCOLATE in its original state. Freshly picked from a cacao tree, chocolate seeds are bitter, super high in antioxidants and full of magnesium. Magnesium helps me poo and helps my body function. Antioxidants keep me young. Raw cacao is a super healing powerful chocolate that is GUILT FREE and HEALING for me. Add 1 teaspoon to hot water and drink as a coffee substitute or yummy warm soothing drink. I may need to add sugar depending on how bitter the chocolate is. If so, I add coconut sugar, maple syrup or stevia.

Add to smoothies, chia pudding, almond mylk and make my own hard chocolates.

RAW OR UNREFINED COCONUT OIL

A really great fat for my brain and my body, that helps pull bad fats out of my body. Use for oil pulling to remove the toxins out of my mouth. Rub on my body as my new skin cream. Add to my hair to lubricate my hair follicles and use instead of hair gel. Heals my gut issues when eaten as it cools my inflammation and soothes my digestive track. I eat 1 teaspoon daily for good gut health.

Use for a mouth cleanser, moisturizer, hair oil, edible fat remover, gut healer and awesome elixir latte maker.

TURMERIC POWDER

I can add on top of all my food and in my salad dressing. Buy the best quality and non radiated brands, so the medicine is fresh. I can also buy turmeric root for making tea and adding to smoothies and juices. Turmeric is very anti-inflammatory so it helps take down the fire in my body. It helps my joints, my aches and pains. The active ingredient is called curcumin and it helps with cancer healing and prevention. Studies show that adding black pepper with the turmeric will bring out the curcumin medicine and make it available for my body to absorb.

FRESH COCONUTS

Drink daily, crack open and eat the meat. Coconut water is 99.9% the same as my human blood. In WWII when they ran out of blood, they used coconut water for blood transfusions as it seamlessly enters our blood stream. Coconut water is very alkaline for my body.

The younger the coconut, the more alkaline the water. Young coconuts have no meat. As the coconut ages, the water gets sweeter and the meat gets thicker. All stages of the coconut are very healthy and I will try all the stages. A very old brown coconut usually has undrinkable water but the meat is amazing for making fresh coconut milk or coconut chips. The fat from the hard meat is used to make coconut oil and is very healthy for my body.

- - ♡ - -

CANS OR CARTONS OF COCONUT MYLK

Coconut mylk sold as cereal milk is usually full of preservatives and weird additives I can't pronounce. Buying canned pure coconut mylk when I can't make my own, is a much better alternative. Once I open the can, I transfer the mylk into a glass jar to get it out of the metal as fast as possible. I can dilute the can with 2 parts water to make mylk for cereals, smoothies or soups. I scoop the thick cream into my smoothies, coffee, teas and hot elixirs. I can also make chia pudding, soups and curry sauces with my coconut mylk. Having coconut mylk in my fridge ready to go all the time, makes food making easy. It is a good fat for my body and for my brain. The fat will help me with my hunger cravings during my JUICY cleanse. I can also now buy pure 100% coconut mylk in littke tetra carton packs that are awesome.

CARTONS OF COCONUT WATER

If I don't have access to fresh, I then buy the best carton brand out there. Read the ingredients as some have preservatives, added chemicals or white sugar. It is great to have cartons of coconut water on hand for my JUICY cleanse. That way if I get hungry or am on the go, I can drink a carton of coconut water and have an instant meal.

SHREDDED COCONUT

I can use shredded coconut to make fresh coconut mylk. I get natural shredded coconut watch out for preservatives in the ingredients. I blend 1 cup of shredded coconut with 2 or 3 cups of warm water to make coconut mylk. I then strain through a nut mylk bag for a yummy fresh coconut mylk. The warm water helps bring the oils out of the coconut meat. Coconut meat is a source of good fat, the kind that pulls bad fat out of my body.

ALMONDS & NUTS

Make fresh nut mylks. Soak my almonds and nuts to clean them and activate their life force. Nuts are dormant until water awakens them. I can soak sunflower sprouts and add them to smoothies and salads, or make dips with them. I can soak cashews to make soups and smoothies creamy, and to make raw desserts. I can soak other nuts to rinse them from the dust or dirt accumulated in bulk bins or plastic bags. I ALWAYS soak almonds. ALWAYS. Almonds in particular have a toxin inside that makes them hard to digest. I put a cup of almonds into 2 cups spring water and leave overnight. In the morning I pour out the toxic sludgy brown water and rinse the almonds. I then eat these activated soft almonds that are easy to digest or I use them to make almond mylk. They taste fresh, like if I picked them off a tree.

PINK HIMALAYAN SALT

For remineralizing my water, salad dressing and adding a pinch to my green juices to bring out their flavor. Pink salt has 72 minerals that are naturally occurring in my body, so when I eat it, I replenish minerals in my body. I eat only really good quality salts and toss out the white stuff. Salt comes from the earth and is a natural substance. White table salt is cooked, processed and is not healthy for my body. White salt causes inflammation inside my body and makes me puffy. Consuming white salt just like sugar, can lead to diabetes. I do need salt for my thrival and I need good quality salt as my body is made up of 80% salt water.

LOOSE LEAF & ROOT TEAS

Tulsy, peppermint, rooibos, matte, green, digestive blends and healing herbs. Using loose leaf is far more superior to tea bagging. Tea bags are usually filled with crumbs left over from loose leaf production. Tea is medicine, so I buy the best quality brands as I want to make sure I ingest the most potent medicine. I can add coconut mylk to make more fatty and filling tea drinks. I blend my hot tea with 1 or 2 tsp of coconut oil in a blender, to make a fatty lattee tea elixir. The coconut oil when blended, will turn into cream and make the best good for me fatty lattee. Vegan style.

CHAGA TEA

Medicinal mushroom tea that helps rebuild my immune system, heals tumours and prevents cancer. Chaga is the tastiest and easiest to brew of the medicinal mushrooms. It tastes like coffee and I can add coconut mylk, to make it extra delicious. Chaga tastes very earthy and most people can feel its effects in their body. It helps boost my immune system and rebuilds me on a cellular level. As I start to ingest the medicinal mushroom family, I start taking my health to the super hero level. I will start playing in a whole new world of eating and healing when I start ingesting these ancient earth wonders. Chaga grows on birch trees and looks like burnt chunks of the tree. Chaga powder or chaga chunks need to be simmered for at least 20 minutes to slowly extract the medicine. I can now find chaga in bioavailable instant powders that only require hot water, rather than cooking. This makes drinking chaga very convenient. I can put hot chaga tea into my blender, add coconut mylk or few teaspoons coconut oil and blend. I will make the most delicious latte and fill my coffee cravings. I can also add coconut sugar when I am not cleansing.

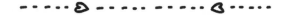

CHAPTER 31

LET'S MAKE
LEMON WATER

L EMONS ARE THE MOST ALKALINE FRUIT on the planet. Seems crazy right? I would think they would the most acidic. When lemons connect with my saliva they turn alkaline, so they are the most powerful way to cleanse and heal my body.

When I sleep, my body is working hard to heal, cleanse and bring me back to my perfect PH balance of acid and alkaline. My body is working for this function 24 hours a day, all the time. So if I feed my body acidic food, then my body has to work extra hard to get me back to my optimal state of alkalinity. Drinking lemon water first thing in the morning, after I have cleansed my mouth, is a routine I can have for the rest of my life.

Lemon water will gently wake up all my organs that have been resting all night. It will alkaline my acidic-on-fire body by reducing the inflammation, reverse premature aging and heal gut rot.

LEMON WATER WILL HEAL ME! So I start it now and do it forever.

Squeeze 1/2 a lemon into a big glass of room temperature spring water (non chlorine, non fluoride, non plastic water) and drink on an empty stomach.

I drink AFTER I have cleansed my mouth – yes I remember!!!

I can also use warm water or sometimes hot water if I am feeling chilly. All variations will help me and the room temperature water will do it the fastest. I follow my intuition and do it the way I like and I DO IT!

I can add slices of ginger and turmeric to my hot lemon water but their medicine is best released by boiling them. I can boil sliced ginger and turmeric roots in water for a few minutes (3-8 min) and add this tea mixture to my lemon water when I want an alteration. Ginger and turmeric are very anti inflammatory and alkalizing for my body

I start with lemon and water first. It is easy and ensures I will do it. And IT WORKS!!!

If I have heart burn or colitis or IBS, I might feel afraid that this drink will burn my already acidic stomach, yet it is completely the opposite. Lemons will heal my stomach over time. I might need to start more gently though, maybe start with a few slices squeezed into water or a few drops of lemon juice in my water. Only I will know what will work for my body and I test it out. I let go of, "this will not work", "my body will not like it" and experiment with my own body and my own healing. I can start using aloe juice to heal my inflamed gut if my body truly is on fire. Aloe juice can be purchased at health food stores or I can filet my own aloe by removing the green plant exterior and blending the slimy gel filet with some water in a blender.

I have the power of my healing IN MY HANDS so I use my time effectively and learn how to heal myself and feel absolutely awesome in my body and super happy in my heart!

An alternative to lemons is RAW apple cider vinegar. Lemons are preferred as they are direct from nature and raw apple cider vinegar is a great second choice. It has to be raw. Bragg's Brand found in healthy grocery stores is the best brand. Add a capful to my glass of water and drink. I can also add to my water bottle for a flavored alkaline drink throughout the day.

Limes, oranges and grapefruits will not have the same alkaline effect like lemons but they do make my water taste delicious and are super healing for my body too. Experiment with adding in as much citrus JUICY food as possible into my life and into my JUICY cleanse. Squeeze ½ orange into my water for a new JUICY water flavor. Make grapefruit water or lime water. Play. This is my JUICY lifestyle I am fulfilling. Science has found that the oil from citrus fruit peels is very anti cancerous and possibly more effective than chemo for many cancers. If my fruit is organic, I put it into my juices and smoothies with the peel.

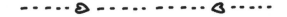

CHAPTER 32

LET'S MAKE GREEN SMOOTHIES

G REENS + FRUIT + WATER + ICE ---> BLEND

Making a green smoothie every morning is a fundamental and impactful part of my JUICY LIFESTYLE! It's the one thing I can add in that will CHANGE my life FOR THE BETTER quickly! I will feel and see the results within a few days. I can create an amazing cleanse by drinking sweet and savory green smoothies through out the day or as my new breakfast routine.

THE BEST PART...

THEY ONLY TAKE **10 MINUTES** TO MAKE!!!

During my JUICY cleanse, I might want to drink juices only or start my mornings off with a green smoothie and then drink juices for the rest of the day. The kind of cleanse I do is up to me and I DO SOMETHING! I can also spend 7 days cutting out an unhealthy food and adding in bowel cleansing and healing green smoothies for my amazing cleanse. The green smoothie will rock my world. I am worth it and my body will be really happy with me!!!!

Green smoothies are now a staple food in my new JUICY lifestyle.

There are many kinds of smoothies I can drink in the morning. GREEN SMOOTHIES are FRUIT smoothies with GREENS added in. Although fruit smoothies are hydrating, they don't do much for my nutritional health as they are mainly sugar that will spike my glycemic levels and then give me a crash. Having a green smoothie is the easiest way to add a bunch of super greens into my diet. It's not often I would eat a few handfuls of spinach or kale for breakfast yet with a green smoothie this is exactly what I do.

It is fun to sip a fruity icy smoothie sometimes but I make it green when ever possible. As part of my JUICY lifestyle, every morning I drink a green smoothie. Some mornings I might forget, some mornings I might get lazy but I just go back to my green smoothie and my body will feel happy again.

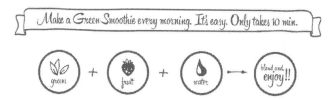

Make a Green Smoothie every morning. It's easy. Only takes 10 min.

greens + fruit + water → blend and enjoy!!

YUMMY SMOOTHIE MAKING TIPS...

- Make as fruity as possible so I want to drink it every morning. I have to love the taste so I want it every morning. If it tastes too green, my taste buds will reject it. Soon I will love it GREENER!

- Use banana as my base fruit. ADD other fruit to mix up the flavors.

- Peel and freeze my bananas for convenience and frosty goodness.

- Always buy fresh greens. Wrap and store greens to maintain freshness. Never freeze my greens, as I want the life force energy to be strong.

- Keep my smoothie pure. Don't add too many extras. Use as a cleansing drink. Too many extra ingredients might slow down my system and be hard to digest. I want this smoothie to give me energy, hydrate and clean me, not be hard work on my body.

A LOVE NOTE FROM PETRA: Once I learned the power of the green smoothie on myself and all those around me, I created *The Green Smoothie Gangster - 40 Day Lifestyle Cleanse* that I teach online and tour around the world. The program is to inspire you to take your health into your hands, lose weight and feell awesome in your body. You can start this gentle cleanse any time and we do it as a group every month. Come join us and let's rock out your life. Doing this 40 Day Cleanse is the fastest way you will notice a difference in your body, your health and your state of mind. Having green smoothies instead of breakfast will change your life I guarantee it.

www.GreenSmoothieGangster.com

40 days to refresh your life with simple food switches, meditation, connection to your body and many other simple practices that will help you feel amazing.

- - ♡ - -

GREEN SMOOTHIE RECIPES...

THE BASE SMOOTHIE RECIPE

2 bananas

3 handfuls spinach

2-3 cups water

Blend together in a BLENDER

- - ♡ - -

CILANTRO, KALE & BANANA

4 leaves kale

1 handful cilantro

1-2 bananas

1 mango

2-3 cups water

Blend together in a BLENDER

- - ♡ - -

BLUEBERRY SMOOTHIE

2 handfuls spinach

3 leaves kale

2 bananas

1 cup blueberries

2-3 cups water

Blend together in a BLENDER

HEMP SEED SMOOTHIE

5 leaves kale

2 tsp. hemp seeds

1 bananas

1 kiwi

2-3 cups water

Blend together in a BLENDER

- - ♥ - -

SPINACH & MANGO SMOOTHIE

2 handfuls spinach

2-3 leaves kale

2 cups mango or 1 cup mango + 1 banana

2-3 cups water

Blend together in a BLENDER

- - ♥ - -

KALE & ORANGE SMOOTHIE

2 handfuls spinach

3 leaves kale

2 bananas

2 oranges freshly squeezed (about 1 cup juice)

1 cup water

Blend together in a BLENDER

- - ♥ - -

CHAPTER 33

LET'S MAKE JUICE

MAKING MY OWN JUICE IS VERY SIMPLE and I can do it. I just need 2 things, a juicing machine and fresh produce.

It is best to come up with a juicing plan for my JUICY cleanse. Juicing usually takes about 1 hour to prep all my veggies, juice them, clean up the juicer and store my juices. So I make some time for myself in the morning.

I make a big jug of juice. I drink 1 or 2 glasses right away and place my leftovers in glass jars in the fridge. I drink this fridge juice as soon as possible too. Juices need to be drank right away as they lose their nutrition and life force. Sometimes I drink it a few hours later or the next day. I know the life force is not as strong, but hey I do what I can for convenience too. If I have a busy life and not have time to make fresh juices 3 times per day, then I can make a big batch of juice first thing in the morning and drink it through out the day.

Having juices ready and on hand will ensure I stick with my JUICY cleanse. When I get hungry, I am able to grab a juice out of my fridge and I stick with my cleanse.

If I am buying juices, I stay away from cold press juice bars that juice the night prior and have juices sitting in the fridge for hours slowly dying. I prefer fresh when possible especially if I am paying for a fresh juice. I ask for it fresh. I am worth it. I always ask for my wheatgrass shots to be juiced right in front of me and I don't buy the pasteurized juices. I ask stores how fresh a juice is and how long it has been sitting in the fridge. I then choose if I want to buy it or not.

To experience what life force tastes like, I create the following experiment. I buy a cold pressed green juice that has been sitting on the shelf for many hours and I buy a freshly pressed green juice. I taste both and choose which one feels more alive and vibrant inside my body. Raw juice sitting a long time in a fridge is still better for me then a pasteurized juice or other processed drinks.

HOW I START MY JUICY CLEANSE?

1. Buy tons of produce. Lots of kale, greens, cucumbers, celery, apples, oranges, beets, carrots, ginger root, turmeric root, lemons, grapefruits, water melon, cabbage, pineapples etc.

2. In the morning wash all the produce I plan to juice.

3. Create two separate juice types. Create a bright color like green, orange or red juice, instead of a muddled brownish color that doesn't seem so appetizing. The brighter the colors, the more my body will want to drink this juice. For example, one will be a green juice and the other will be a red juice.

4. Chop my green batch first and let it soak in a kitchen sink to absorb some water, rinse and perk up my greens. Add a splash of white vinegar to the soaking water to kill any possible germs. Chop green leaves, cucumbers, apples or oranges, lemons, ginger, turmeric and a little celery. Celery will take over the flavor of my juice so I use only a little or make a separate celery only juice. Celery juice is very healing, full of the perfect salt water to rehydrate my cells.

5. Place all my chopped produce into a big bowl and start juicing. Mix the leaves with hard apples or carrots to push the fiber through the juicer. Sometimes too many greens will clog the juicer and this sucks as I will have to dissemble and clean the juicer to continue.

6. Pour all my green juice through a sieve or strainer to remove any excess pulp fiber for taste purposes. If I like pulp floating in my juice then I don't have to do this step. Some juicers will give me clean juice and some will not fully strain out the pulp so I can do this extra step.

7. Pour all my strained juice into glass jars and drink a BIG glass right away, or a few glasses while it is fresh and full of life force. I then place the rest of the jars in the fridge for the rest of the day.

8.   Next I prep and juice my red or orange batch of juice. I chop and soak beets, carrots, oranges or grapefruits, watermelon, cabbage, ginger, turmeric, etc. I repeat steps 5 - 8.

My juice produce combinations are up to me. The less fruit I use, the healthier my juice will be. If I am healing from cancer or sickness, I then reduce or remove all fruit and just use lemons for flavour so I am not adding sugar into my system. Adding fruit does make my juice taste yummy, so I use enough fruit to break the veggie taste, without making a sugary drink.

Celery has quite a distinct taste and can make all my juices taste similar when I add it. I use celery sparingly and try making my juice combinations with and without celery so I can taste the difference. Celery is full of water and good for me salt. Drinking straight up celery juice is very healthy for me too. So again, I play with my juicing combinations and create juices I love and that are super healthy for me. I am brave, clever and I can do this. I can be a juicing cleansing master in no time.

The following is a guide of ingredient combinations I can play with. I need to add fruit or citrus to break the green veggie taste.

RED OR ORANGE JUICE INGREDIENTS

beets
red cabbage
carrots
ginger root
turmeric root

Add citrus or fruit to red or orange juice
lemons
apples
grapefruits
oranges
limes
watermelon
pineapples

- - ♡ - -

GREEN JUICE INGREDIENTS
green leaves (kale, cilantro, spinach, romaine lettuce,
parsley, collards, dandelion, etc)
cucumbers
celery
green herbs (mint, basil, etc)
fennel root
green cabbage
asparagus
ginger and turmeric root

Add citrus or fruit to green juice:
lemons
apples
oranges
pineapples
grapefruit
limes

JUICY RECIPES...

PETRA'S GREEN JUICE
(chopped big bowl of produce)
green leaves – kale, cilantro, spinach, bok choy, romaine
wheatgrass if i want
lemons
cucumbers
apples
pineapples
few carrots
ginger root
turmeric root

- - ♥ - -

PETRA'S RED JUICE
(chopped big bowl of produce)
beets
watermelon
grapefruit
red cabbage
few carrots
limes
ginger root
turmeric root

PETRA'S ORANGE JUICE

(chopped big bowl of produce)

carrots

oranges

apples

ginger root

turmeric root

- - ♥ - -

CANTALOUPE JUICE

2 cantaloupes

GREEN it - add cilantro or spinach / kale

* Filling and creamy

- - ♥ - -

CARROT APPLE LEMON JUICE

6 carrots

3 apples

3 celery stalks

1 head romaine lettuce

1 lemon

GREEN it - add spinach / kale

* Juice up your cells

LEMON APPLE JUICE

6 apples

1 lemon

GREEN it – add cilantro / spinach / kale

* Great for breaking kidney stones

- - ♡ - -

PINEAPPLE STRAWBERRY JUICE

1 pineapple keeping middle stem (peeled)

8 strawberries with stem

GREEN it – add romain lettuce

* Great brain food

- - ♡ - -

WATERMELON BEETJUICE

peel and juice watermelon

add 1 or 2 beets

add lime or mint

GREEN it – add spinach / kale

* Alkaline and hydrate your body

* Great bowel cleanser

LIME ORANGE JUICE

5 oranges

1 lime

GREEN it – add cilantro / spinach / kale

* Great source of calcium

- - ♡ - -

APPLE ORANGE CARROT JUICE

4 apples

4 oranges

8 carrots

GREEN it – add cilantro / spinach / kale

* Enhance your vision and get skin glow

- - ♡ - -

APPLE KIWI JUICE

3 apples

3 oranges

3 kiwis

GREEN it – add cilantro / spinach

* Boost your vitamin C like crazy

CELERY KALE JUICE

6 carrots

4 celery stalks

4 leaves kale

2 apples

1 lime

* Green and alkalize you up

- - ♡ - -

CUCUMBER CILANTRO APPLE JUICE

1 cucumber

3 apples

3 celery stalks

1 bunch cilantro

* Get the glow

- - ♡ - -

APPLE GINGER JUICE

6 apples

medium piece ginger

GREEN it – add cilantro / spinach / kale

* Keep the doctor away and break kidney stones

APPLE BEET JUICE

4 apples

1 beet

1 lime

GREEN it – add cilantro / spinach / kale

* Clean you out

- - ♡ - -

PINEAPPLE KALE JUICE

1/4 fresh pineapple skin removed

4 leaves kale

1/2 lime

1 nub ginger

* Use core of pineapple, has high amount
bromelain which is brain food

- - ♡ - -

APPLE KALE JUICE

4 apples

4 leaves kale

1 bunch cilantro

1/2 lime

1 nub ginger

GREEN JUICE

1 bunch kale
1 bunch cilantro
1 bunch collards
1/2 bunch parsley
4 apples
1 lime

- - ♡ - -

YOU CAN DO THIS

GO FOR IT!

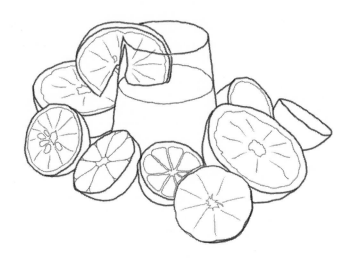

CHAPTER 34

LET'S DRINK WATER

D O I DRINK ENOUGH WATER? Most of the time I probably don't. Most likely, I can go a whole day and realize I drank hardly any water.

Drinking water is a practice. Yes a practice. That means I keep doing it and practicing it. If I forget, that's ok. I will remember again and pick up the glass of water and drink it. It's that simple. During this JUICY cleanse, I drink lots of water in between my juices so I continue flushing my body. The more water and liquids I drink, the more I will flush.

At the stem of most sickness is dehydration. When my cells are not getting hydrated enough, they shrivel up and prematurely die. Some doctors are quoted as saying, "you are not sick, you are dehydrated." I keep my cells JUICY and hydrated so that they remain healthy and I remain young.

My body is 80% water and as I get older, I begin to dry up. I am born a juicy grape and I will die as a shriveled raison unless I keep up my juiciness.

Drinking water is such an important part of my life and where my water comes from is even more important.

What kind of water am I drinking? Is it full of fluoride and chlorine? Is it recycled and cleaned toilet water? Is it living in plastic leaching containers? Is it dead or is it alive?

What kind of water is my life blood made from? And am I willing to up level myself starting right now?

Getting water from a reliable source is super important. Spring water has been naturally filtered and processed through the earth and when it is ready for human consumption, it emerges out of the ground and forms into a natural spring. Spring water comes from aquifers, which are massive lakes in the center of the earth. As rain water falls, the earth absorbs the water, purifies it and fills up its water reserve aquifers. Then as this water percolates and purifies even further, it eventually gains levitational energy and travels up all the layers of the earth to emerge as a raw alive active living life force spring water.

The longest living civilizations and villages formed around natural springs because people knew spring water is life. Most springs form small ponds or have a pipe added, to access the water. Spring water is running and is constantly fresh.

To find a spring in my area, I can check out this website www.findaspring.com, Google local springs or delivery companies in my local community.

Bottled water is a terrible trend that has erupted and made a lot of corporations, especially Coke and Pepsi, a lot of money. It has created so much plastic in landfills and there are giant islands of plastic bottles on the ocean. Plastic bottles are made of unsafe plastic that leach chemicals into the water especially if they sit in the sun or the heat. These chemicals mess with people's hormones, are cancer causing and increase estrogen levels in men and women. Most plastic water is bottled tap water that has been filtered.

Tap water in most cities has fluoride added to it. I have been brainwashed to believe that fluoride is good for my teeth. Fluoride is super toxic, is stored in rooms with hazard signs and workers who handle it have to wear full body hazmat suits so they don't come into contact with this toxic substance. Research says, fluoride was first introduced to the human population by Hitler in WWII, as it calcifies the pineal gland. My pineal glad is in the center of my forehead and is where I connect to my intuition and to my sovereign soul. Hitler knew that people with calcified and shut down pineal glands would be more docile, be better followers and not stand up for their rights.

Tap water also has chlorine added to it with the belief that it prevents mold or bacteria getting into the water. This is also unnecessary as spring water is pure and does not have bacteria living in it. Ozonating water with an Ozone machine will naturally kill any bad bacteria and still be healing for the body. Over time ingesting chlorine kills the good bacteria in my stomach and lowers my immune system. This makes my body susceptible for disease as my body is no longer equipped to handle anything that comes at it. New research shows that chlorine interference is at the stem of cancers and major illnesses due to how much it interrupts the natural system of the body. Tests have been done showing children doing simple math in a small room. Then those same children TRYING to do simple math after the room has been washed with bleach (chlorine). Their brains cannot function and their clarity is gone.

Big cities without access to a fresh water source, clean and recycle sewage water and give it back to the people as tap drinking water. Some cities have to filter the water over 8 times to remove the sewage taste. So any chemicals, pharmaceutical pills, recreational drugs, antibiotics, steroids and garbage people have in their systems stays in the "cleaned" tap water and gets re drank by the people. In some cities, tap water can be more harmful, then good.

Alkalized water created by an alkalizer machine like Kangen for example, is great especially when cleansing or healing disease. The fastest way for me to heal is to get my body to an alkaline state and drink super alkaline water. Most alkalizing machines are quite expensive and are still using tap water as their base.

So the healthiest way to get clean water is to go right to the earth source and collect my own spring water. Spring water is alive and full of life force energy. It is perfectly molecularly structured for my body to understand so it hydrates me instantly. It is the fastest way to flush my body with mass hydration and to connect me to the natural rhythms of the earth. When I start drinking earth water, I get grounded to the earth. My body begins to beat at the natural pulse of the earth energy and this is very healing. My modern world full of radioactive electronics has disconnected me from the vibration of the earth and hence I can get sick and unsettled. The earth is here to support me and to make sure I am a thriving human on this planet. When I drink earth water, my body goes back into alignment with the healing earth energy rhythms.

WAYS I CAN ADD MORE WATER TO MY JUICY LIFESTYLE...

1. EAT RAW FOOD - It's full of water and lots of oxygen too. My body needs lots of water and oxygen to heal, cleanse, flush, lose weight and look younger. The more water and oxygen I can add to my body, the faster my body heals. So I add as much raw juicy food into my new JUICY lifestyle and hydrate! Eating only raw food for a week is also a great way to cleanse.

    What is raw food? It is leafy greens, nuts, seeds, vegetables, fruit, medicinal mushrooms, algae, super foods and good fats like avocado, coconut oil, olive oil, flax oil, hemp oil, nut oils and seed butters, in their natural state. Raw food is full of life force as it has not been cooked or pasteurized. Eating raw food will give me TONS of energy and vitality. I will thrive on a raw food diet if I concentrate on greens, good fats, juicy fruit, super foods and blending everything up. I don't eat too many nuts and seeds as they might be harder to digest and slow my body down.

An amazing cleanse for me could be to add more and more raw food into my lifestyle and commit to eating mainly raw food for 5 days and see how I feel. This powerful food will help me clean and heal my body. From now on, I switch out as much cooked food for raw food and watch my body transform.

2. WAKE AND DRINK - Upon waking AFTER cleaning my mouth, I drink a big glass of water. Could be my lemon water drink or even before my lemon water, I can drink a glass of spring water. In the morning my body wants to flush out. It wants to go poo a few times, but if I don't give my body enough liquid in the morning, it cannot do this simple task. Imagine that I have a few poos in my system lined up and ready to come out. If I drink enough liquid in the morning, this elimination will happen. If I do not, I will carry my poos around with me all day. Hee hee hee! Funny visual.

3. ADD ESSENTIAL OILS - 100% pure edible oils are wonderful for adding into my water to change up the flavor and add plant medicine into my body. Best edible brands are *Young Living* and *Do Terra*. Some brands of oils can have as little as 1% oil and still be considered an essential oil. So I buy the purest oils as they are medicine. I can replace most of my medicine cabinet and beauty regimes with essential oils.

Some oils I can add to my water are: Orange, Lemon, Lime, Peppermint, Lavender, Grapefruit, Frankincense, and Cilantro. These companies have warehouses world wide, so I can get my oils no matter where I live. I can sign up as a full member to get whole sale pricing and get bonus oils or buy retail. I can also find a rep in my community and order through them.

4. FLAVOR MY WATER – I can flavor my water with fruit and leafy herbs to make delicious refreshing JUICY drinks. It is easiest to use a blender to create my JUICY water masterpieces. The amount of fruit is minimal because I am just slightly flavoring my water. This is not a smoothie, it is fruit flavoring for my water.

JUICY BERRY YUM
4 cups water
½ cup raspberries or strawberries
few mint leaves
ice
* BLEND

- - ♡ - -

JUICY CITRUS YUM
4 cups water
¼ cup lemon slices
¼ cup lime slices
few basil leaves
* BLEND

JUICY MANGO YUM

4 cups water
½ cup mango few chunks
few mint leaves
ice
* BLEND

- - ♥ - -

JUICY PINEAPPLE YUM

4 cups water
½ cup pineapple
few mint leaves
ice
* BLEND

- - ♥ - -

5. GET A JUG – I get a big water bottle, ideally a 3 quart / 3 liter size jug made from glass or a good quality plastic. I fill it every morning and drink all of it by the end of the day. Having a marker of how much I drink throughout the day, can be helpful as most likely when I get busy, I forget to drink. Even better if I can fill this jug up several times throughout my day as I am hydrating myself. Sometimes drinking enough water just comes down to accessibility and having my water sitting right beside me. When I visually see it and when I have a goal, I will drink it.

A LOVE NOTE FROM PETRA: I am a huge fan of drinking spring water and have been drinking only spring water for the past 10 + years. I collect my own as I travel the world or find companies that can deliver the bottled spring water to me. I rarely buy bottled water unless I am flying or in some emergency. I carry a refillable jug in my purse at all times or in my car when I live in the Western World. I believe in the power of spring water with all my being and know this is one of the fastest ways to healing and grounding to the frequency of the earth. My body is made up of unprocessed activated earth water and I feel really good about that. Some of the longest living people created their villages around springs and my super hero level health friends all drink spring water too. We are a tribe of people all over the world who drink only spring water and believe in its magic. Wanna join us?

Fresh clean water is our birth right as humans and animals on this planet. We should not be relying on plastic store bought water for our survival. If something happens and the stores run out of water, what will we drink? We have allowed corporations to control our water sources and it is time for us to take this power back. You with me?

The easiest way to take our power back is to go collect our water from the purest source, our mother earth. It is also time for us to speak up to government and public officials to open up our spring water sources, as many have had concrete poured over them. The earth should give us our water, not Coke or Pepsi. Please stop supporting these corrupt corporations and stop buying their plastic water. Please stop buying plastic bottled water forever! Go find a spring near you and go into nature to collect your water, or find a company that will deliver this magic elixir to you.

You are worth it...and so am I. Love You...Petra

- - ♡ - -

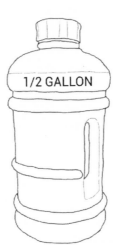

1/2 GALLON

CHAPTER 35

LET'S MAKE NUT MYLK

MOST STORE BOUGHT ALMOND MYLKS have less than 3% almonds or some have none at all. Usually it is a chemical concoction that they call almond mylk. So I learn how to make my own and stop putting these excess preservatives into my body. It is very simple and quick to make my own almond mylk or any nut mylk I desire.

I will be able to taste my homemade mylk, compare it to the flavor of the store bought carton kind and notice the big difference.

There are many non dairy mylks on the market today, so I have a lot of options to never drink dairy milk again. Most are sold in cartons and found on the shelves or fridge isles of my grocery store. I read the ingredients of everything and then chose accordingly. I avoid soy mylk as most soy is genetically modified and the soy bean is owned by Monsanto (aka the devil). Soy is an allergen to my body and causes allergic reactions when eaten. Most of these store bought mylks will be acidic to my body and I should only drink them sparingly (if at all).

A delicious alternative to making my own mylk or buying the carton cereal kind (which has a lot of chemicals), is to buy canned coconut mylk found in the ethnic sections of grocery stores and now also found in little carton packages. This is 100% pure coconut mylk with no added fillers except usually a preservative. Although it is sitting in a can, it will be healthier for my body then the carton brands that have many ingredients. I can use the canned mylk to add cream to my coffee, smoothies and also dilute with water to make mylk for cereals. I dilute 1 can to 2 cans of water, or less depending on the creaminess I want.

Upon opening my canned mylk, I transfer it to a glass jar right away. I avoid cans as much as possible as I don't want to add metals to my body. If I am blessed to live in tropical climates where I can get fresh coconuts, I make my own coconut mylk. Yummy!!!! This is quite a delicacy!

When making my own nut mylk, I use 1 part nuts to 2 or 3 parts water, depending on how creamy I want it. I can use almonds, brazil nuts, cashews and shredded coconut to make awesome mylks. I can also make hemp mylk, which is the easiest because I don't need to strain the seeds from the mylk. Hemp seeds dissolve in the water. A few table spoons of hemp seeds mixed with 2 cups water makes a simple mylk too. Hemp seeds are quite strong in taste, so I use a smaller amount to get used to the taste. I can add a little coconut sugar and vanilla to make my delicious high protein mylks.

NUTS I CAN TO USE FOR MYLK...

Almonds
Brazil nuts
Cashews
Hemp seeds
Dry shredded coconut meat
Fresh hard coconut meat

SOAKING MY NUTS...

Almonds are a must to soak overnight as they contain an enzyme inhibitor that prevents them from growing into an almond tree, is quite toxic and hard to digest. Never reuse the almond soaking water, instead toss it. All other nuts do not need to be soaked and can make mylk instantly, but will blend up better when they are soaked.

To soak my almonds, place 1 cup nuts into jar with 2 cups water and leave overnight. In the morning my soaking water will be brown and sludgy, I toss it out. I rinse off my almonds and now they are ready to use for mylk or to snack on. I will notice my almonds have sponged up a lot of water and are most likely double their size. They will taste soft like they have been freshly picked off a tree and are much easier for my body to digest. They make a great munching snack too.

MAKING ALMOND MYLK...

1 cup soaked overnight almonds, drained and washed

3 cups water

* Blend in blender

* Pour through nut mylk bag

* Strain it and squeeze it

* Toss out pulp

* Drink my fresh mylk

Add: Vanilla or maple syrup or raw cacao to yum it up

Tip: Use 1 or 2 cups water instead for creamier and thicker

Tip: Soak other nuts also. Dont soak shredded coconut

- - ♥ - -

GOLDEN MYLK

1 cup soaked overnight almonds drained and washed

3 cups water

1 finger of turmeric

3 tsp. coconut sugar

Few dashes black pepper

* Blend in blender

* Pour through nut mylk bag.

* Strain and squeeze

* Toss out pulp

Optional: Add cardamom, clove, cinnamon

ORANGE MYLK

2 cups already made mylk
1 squeezed orange
1 tsp. coconut sugar

* Blend in blender
* Drink my fresh mylk

- - ♡ - -

MANGO MYLK

2 cups already made mylk
½ mango

* Blend in blender
* Drink my fresh mylk

- - ♡ - -

CHOCOLATE MYLK

2 cups already made mylk
2 tsp. raw cacao
3 tsp. coconut sugar

* Blend in blender
* Drink my fresh mylk

CHOCOLATE MINT MYLK

2 cups already made mylk

2 tsp. raw cacao

3 tsp. coconut sugar

1 drop peppermint edible essential oil

* Blend in blender
* Drink my fresh mylk

- - ♡ - -

BERRY MYLK

2 cups already made mylk

¼ cup berries

1 tsp. coconut sugar

* Blend in blender
* Drink my fresh mylk

- - ♡ - -

HEMP MYLK

2 tbsp. hemp seeds

2 cups water

* Blend and drink my fresh mylk
* Don't need to strain as hemp seeds dissolve

Add: Vanilla or maple syrup or raw cacao to yum it up

CHAPTER 36

LET'S MAKE RAW SOUP

R AW SOUPS ARE A PERFECT FILLER FOOD for my JUICY cleanse and an awesome addition to my JUICY lifestyle. They are raw, full of life force, nutrition and are similar to a smoothie but a bit more filling and satiating.

Drinking creamy RAW soups can help ease me into my JUICY cleanse. If I want a gentler start to my cleanse, then I add them to the first few days. They will fill me up and my digestion will still get a break, as they are liquid.

A great way to UP LEVEL my already cooked soups, is to put the hot soup into my blender, add dark leafy RAW greens and blend everything together. Now I have a hot soup that has green raw super power inside. Great for pumpkin soup or any veggie soup that I want to add more nutrition, vitamins and life force. I will notice a difference in my body when I eat a fully cooked soup and when I eat a fully raw or ½ raw soup. I will feel more life force energy inside my body. I can also add other raw vegetables to hot soups, like carrots, tomatoes, broccoli, beets, ginger, turmeric and blend everything in the blender. If I have children, this is also a powerful way to add raw nutrition to their diet without them knowing it. "Thank you soup.... You make me happy in my tummy!"

RAW SOUP RECIPES...

Add 1/4 cup soaked overnight cashews, mac nuts, hemp seeds or ½ avocado to add more fat and make my soups creamy.

SPINACH RAW SOUP
2 cups spinach
1 tomato
½ peeled cucumber
1 avocado
2 cups hot water OR some coconut mylk
2 tbsp. wheat free tamari (soy sauce)
½ tsp. salt
1 tsp. chopped ginger
1 tbsp. lemon juice
dash cayenne and pepper
½ tsp. turmeric

* Blend in BLENDER until smooth and creamy

KALE RAW SOUP

2 cups fresh almond or coconut mylk
1 tbsp. lemon juice
½ avocado
3-5 leaves kale
handful cilantro (optional)
1 clove garlic
1 green onion
1 tbsp. nutritional yeast flakes
½ tsp. salt
½ tsp. turmeric
dash black pepper

* Blend in BLENDER until smooth and creamy

- - ♥ - -

AWESOME MISO RAW SOUP

pour 2 cups warm / hot water into blender
add 2 tbsp. miso
add green onion, garlic, salt or other spices I desire

* Blend and drink
* Miso is a mineral rich broth full of alive nutrients
* Miso is a simple and AWESOME way to make instant food
* Ideally buy soy free healthy version miso paste from an
organic grocery store
* Never cook or boil miso, add to hot water after stove
turned off or into blender

INSTANT MISO SOUP

1 tsp. miso paste in mug

1 cup hot water

* Put miso in mug and add ½ cup water
* Stir to blend
* Add remaining hot water
* Stir and drink
* AWESOME snack for the office
* Bring a jar of miso with me to work and store in fridge
* Make when I feel hungry or want something salty and yummy

- - ♡ - -

PETRA'S SIMPLE RAW HOT CLEANSING SOUP

few handfuls dark leafy greens

(mix of: kale, spinach, beet tops, cilantro, parsley, bok choy)

few cherry tomatoes

½ avocado or ½ cup soaked cashews

½ squeezed lemon

salt

pepper

cayenne or chili spice

few cups hot water

* Blend in blender
* Can add onions, garlic, ginger
* Can be made into a savory smoothie using cold water
* Great soup for cleaning out my fridge and throwing in bits
of left over veggies to experiment

CHAPTER 37

LET'S TALK FAT

THERE IS A LOT OF INFORMATION OUT THERE about fats and proteins. Is eating fats good for me or bad for me? How do I know which fats to eat? Marketing has tried to brain wash me to believe that fat is bad for me and I should consume low fat or no fat foods. This ridiculous campaign has added to the obesity of people and increase in sickness, perhaps even in myself.

I stop being scared of FAT and automatically thinking FAT will make me FAT! It depends on the type of fat I am eating, as my body needs healthy fat to thrive.

Good fats pull bad fats out of my body. It is important for me to eat good fats to feed my brain, my organs and my muscles. My brain is made of fat. I need fat as a part of my JUICY lifestyle. A diet consisting primarily of greens, veggies and healthy fats is my optimal eating. I add in some fruits, nuts, seeds, seaweeds and super foods and I am rocking my JUICY lifestyle. During my JUICY cleanse, I may want to cut fats out completely and just stick with fresh juices and fresh smoothies. Or I may start out with some fatty smoothies, soups and nut mylks to ease my way into juices only. How I choose to cleanse is up to me.

FATS FOR MY SMOOTHIES...

I can add these fats to my green or mylky smoothies. I experiment with what I like and always keep the green smoothie as simple as possible for cleansing and optimal health. Add fatty mylky smoothies to my cleanse for more sustenance and for a variety of liquid food I can eat any time of the day. Food in a blender is easy and quick food. It makes my JUICY lifestyle easy and is awesome for on going every day simple cleansing.

CHOOSE 1 OR A COMBINATION TO ADD TO MY SMOOTHIES...

2 tbsp. hemp seeds
2 tbsp. chia seeds
½ avocado
2 tbsp. almond butter
2 tbsp. coconut oil
2 tbsp. coconut butter
2 tbsp. canned coconut mylk
1 whole coconut water + meat
2 tbsp. MCT oil
2 tbsp. flax oil
2 tbsp. hemp oil

CHAPTER 38

LET'S TALK PROTEIN

HAVE ALSO BEEN BRAINWASHED ABOUT the proteins to add to my smoothies. Soy protein and whey protein are not good for me and cause inflammation in my body and are allergens to my body. This means my body has to work hard to process them as it sees them as harmful invaders.

Over the past several years amazing raw plant based proteins have emerged on the market. Plant based protein is instantly assimilated by my body and gives my body extra energy instead of hard work. It is made from whole food so it is full of nutrients, vitamins and life force.

I have also been brainwashed about what protein to eat for my meals and led to believe that I have to eat meat in order for my body to receive a good source of protein. Meat protein is very acidic to my body and very hard for my body to digest. When it is cooked, it loses all its digestive enzymes needed to digest the meat. Carnivorous animals eat their meat raw and usually eat alkaline bones with their meal. Their intestines are very short and this raw meat digests through their body quickly. I am not this carnivorous animal, my teeth and my body are not designed to eat meat, especially when it is cooked.

Some of the biggest and strongest animals on the planet do not eat meat for their protein, they eat GREEN PLANTS. Gorillas, elephants, horses and cows eat green food for their protein and they are extremely strong. I have been brainwashed to believe that I must eat a cow for my protein, but I am actually getting my protein from the green food the cow has eaten. I am eating the processing machine rather than eating plant based protein right from its source.

Green leaves and dark green vegetables are extremely high in protein and are alkaline for my body. They are full of chlorophyll which is the same as my own blood and they clean my body with every bite. So making a green smoothie every morning with lots of spinach and kale, gives my body protein.

PROTEIN FOR MY SMOOTHIES...

I can add these proteins to my mylky and green smoothies. I keep my green smoothies as pure as possible so they give me instant healing energy. My body doesn't have to work very hard to process greens and fruit. I experiment with what proteins I like and make sure I am choosing pure plant based sources of protein for my body to feel happy. Some plant based protein powders have soy and other fillers, so I read the ingredients of everything before I buy it.

CHOOSE 1 OR A COMBINATION TO ADD TO MY SMOOTHIES...

2 tbsp. hemp seeds
2 tbsp. chia seeds
2 tbsp. almond butter
2 tbsp. coconut butter
¼ cup soaked and rinsed almonds
¼ cup cashews
¼ cup sunflower seeds
¼ cup pumpkin seeds
¼ cup brazil nuts
2 tbsp. hemp protein powder
2 tbsp. sun warrior rice protein powder
2 tbsp. any raw plant based protein powder

PETRA'S GOING RAW SMOOTHIE

1 Thai young coconut water + meat
2 tbsp. hemp seeds
2 tbsp. raw cacao powder
1-2 tbsp. coconut sugar

* Crack open coconut using coco jack tool
* Pour liquid into blender
* Scoop out all white fleshy meat with a big spoon into blender
* Add all other ingredients
* Blend and drink
* Use stevia, maple syrup or dates as other ways to sweeten

A LOVE NOTE FROM PETRA: 12 years ago, when I first went raw, my boyfriend and I would make this GOING RAW SMOOTHIE every morning together as our routine. We would crack open a coconut with a giant butcher knife in our Vancouver apartment kitchen. This was before my Maui coconut cracking jungle days and before I discovered green smoothies.

I LOVED this smoothie for so many reasons and now, for my body, it is too heavy in the morning. I now prefer starting my day with a green smoothie, green juice or coconut water instead. Try it for yourself though as it is a great transition food into your JUICY lifestyle and liquid cleansing routines.

Get this new easy coconut opening tool at www. coco-jack.com. It will make your life so much easier and way less dangerous than a butcher knife like we used. Lucky we never got hurt.

- - ♡ - -

CHAPTER 39

LET'S MAKE A KICKASS SALAD

DO I KNOW HOW TO MAKE A KICK ASS JUICY salad? Yummy, huge, awesome, full of goodies, big bowl of salad that will make me full and energized after eating.

Salads can be a great way to ease into my JUICY cleanse by having them in the first few days along with my juices and smoothies. After a few days, I can transition to liquids only, so my body no longer has to do any digesting. Replacing one meal in my day with a kickass salad can also be a great way to cleanse and heal my body as a much slower and longer process.

Maybe I've had a bad view of salads and have never craved to eat them. Most restaurants have LAME salads with only a few ingredients. There's not much sustenance to them. A typical standard American salad is head lettuce, a few tomatoes and cucumber slices with a very crappy, terrible for me salad dressing on top. It is no wonder most people cringe at the sound of a salad. They sound and taste so boring that no one wants to order them.

A lot of restaurants serve wilted green salads, using boxed or bagged not so fresh greens that are lacking LIFEFORCE! I might order a salad because I crave a lighter meal or want to make healthy choices but the lack of nutrients in the produce makes my salad eating experience nothing to write home about. I might leave the restaurant and soon be hungry again and feel it was a waste of money.

So it is time to CHANGE how I view, eat and think about SALADS! It is time to make kickass salads that make my mouth salivate and leave me craving my next bowl. A kickass salad is perfect for breakfast, lunch or dinner and makes the perfect packed lunch. If I prep my ingredients ahead of time, it can be the fastest dinner I throw together when I get home tired from work. Kickass salads are awesome and energizing. They will become my new best friend, along with the green smoothie for my new JUICY lifestyle and cleansing experience.
Most important is I want to feel excited to eat it, so I make it yummy!!!! This is a good for me food that tastes really good too.

Am I planning to eat salads on my JUICY cleanse or am I sticking to liquids only and no digesting for 1 week? Or am I cleansing with liquids and 1 salad meal per day? The level of cleansing is really up to me. I can drink green smoothies, juices and eat salads throughout the day and HAVE THE MOST INCREDIBLE cleanse ever. I go for it and do what feels right for my body. I am BRAVE to let go of chewing and digesting for 1 week to heal and reboot my body. It takes guts to do a JUICY cleanse and I am super proud of me.

For my upcoming new JUICY lifestyle, I can eat in a way that is a gentle cleanse every day. I can continue eating food that is healing and cleaning the old garbage out of my body. So once I finish my JUICY cleanse and move into my JUICY lifestyle, then green smoothies and kickass green salads are part of my new lifestyle routine.

If I am eating salad as part of my JUICY cleanse, then I limit the amount of oil I use in my dressing and maybe even just use lemon juice or apple cider vinegar with a few drops of oil to break down the greens. The less oil, the more I will cleanse.

PREP THE NIGHT BEFORE...

I create my kickass big salad the night before I go to work. Put dressing into a separate container and pour on when I am ready to eat. Take my salad with me on the go and have an amazing nutritious, energizing and filling meal that will make me feel super JUICY!

I can also prep by chopping all my veggies and putting them into separate containers in the fridge. That way when I am hungry, I have fast food on hand and can quickly make a salad. I will cheat on my JUICY cleanse, if when I get hungry, I grab crappy food for convenience. To ensure my success, I have to have ingredients ready and accessible.

KICKASS SALAD GREENS

kale

spinach

collards

romaine lettuce

baby lettuce

bok choy

cilantro

parsley

sunflower sprouts

* Avoid head lettuce as it has no nutritional value

- - ♡ - -

KICKASS SALAD VEGGIES

avocado - chopped

cucumber - chopped

carrot – grated

celery – chopped

beet – grated

radish – chopped

broccoli – chopped

cauliflower - chopped

cabbage – sliced thin

onions - chopped

peas - fresh or canned

corn – fresh or canned (harder for body to digest)

KICKASS DRESSING INGREDIENTS

raw apple cider vinegar

raw sauerkraut juice

olive oil

avocado oil

hemp oil

flax oil

himalayan pink salt

hemp seeds

avocado

lemons

limes

spices

nutritional yeast

almond butter

raw maple syrup

coconut

coconut sugar

dates

garlic

onions

jalapenos

- - ♡ - -

KICKASS SALAD TOPPINGS

pumpkin seeds

sesame seeds

hemp seeds

spirulina powder

jalepeno peppers

dried flaky seaweed

dates, raisons, apricots – chopped small

nuts – chopped small

nutritional yeast

hummus

raw sauerkraut

mango

peaches

blueberries

strawberries

If I buy salad dressing from a grocery store, I make sure I read the ingredients first. If it is made with canola oil or some vegetable oil other than olive oil, I don't buy it. Canola oil was never meant for human consumption and is a machine oil. It is harmful for my body and is a bad fat for me. I only buy pure olive oil salad dressings or MAKE MY OWN!!!

It is simple to make a few ingredient salad dressing. I can combine OIL + SOUR + SALT + WATER. Always add water so I don't have to use too much oil to make my base. I use healthy vinegars or citrus fruits for my sour and natural mineral salt.

Here are a few ideas for making my own dressings. Simple is better and much easier. I can make any combination of healing magic I wish. As long as I am using healthy healing ingredients, then I can play to make my FAVORITE dressing recipes. I buy good quality oils like pumpkin, avocado, walnut, hemp, flax or good quality olive oil. Oil is medicine and I make sure I put a good healing fat into my body.

SALAD DRESSING RECIPES...

SIMPLE DRESSING A
raw apple cider vinegar + olive oil + Himalayan pink salt

- - ♡ - -

SIMPLE DRESSING B
raw sauerkraut juice + olive oil + Himalayan pink salt

- - ♡ - -

SIMPLE DRESSING C
dressing A or B + avocado

* Mix in blender

SIMPLE DRESSING D

dressing A + hemp seeds, spices, lemon or lime and almond
butter

* Mix in blender

- - ♥ - -

SIMPLE DRESSING E

dressing A + nutritional yeast, turmeric powder, black pepper,
salt, tamari wheat free soy sauce

* Mix in blender

- - ♥ - -

CHAPTER 40

LET'S MAKE CHIA PUDDING

C HIA PUDDING IS AN EASY SNACK FOR ME to make for myself that is high in protein, good fats and gives me that yogurt / pudding experience without any dairy, chemical crap or harm to animals. Chia pudding also has maximum nutrients with minimal calories.

Chia seeds are high in omega 3 oils, they turn gelatinous when wet, they have lots of protein and are a good source of chlorophyll. Because they get gelatinous, much like aloe gel, they are amazing for healing my digestive track as they cool and sooth my inner fire. They also slowly expand in my belly, giving me a more full feeling longer when I eat them in smoothies, as pudding or sprinkled on cereals. When they are planted, chia seeds will sprout to little green nutritious plants.

In the early 80s, before chia seeds were in our food supply, they were sold as chia pets. If I had a chia pet, I would soak the seeds and spread the gelatinous mixture on a terra cota statue and the chia seeds would turn into fuzzy green plant hair. All of a sudden, my chia pet would be furry. Now instead of spreading on statues, society recognizes chia seeds as the super food they are.

Making chia pudding is simple and quick. I can eat it instantly or wait for my mixture to thicken. I use chia pudding in the place of yogurt and sugar pudding. I can use chia seeds to make parfaits, puddings, smoothies, sprinkle on fruit, add to cereal, mix in flavored water or add to juices.

VANILLA CHIA PUDDING

1 cup coconut mylk or other nut mylk
2 tbsp. chia seeds
few drops or ½ tsp. vanilla
2 tbsp. maple syrup

* Stir in glass jar
* Place in fridge
* Leave 20 or more minutes
* Eat

Tip: If I use coconut sugar, then it's best to blend the mylk and sugar in a blender first, then add the chia seeds in the jar. The sugar will dissolve much better.

PINEAPPLE CHIA PUDDING

1 cup coconut mylk or other nut mylk
½ cup chopped pineapple
2 tbsp. chia seeds
2 tbsp. maple syrup or 1 tbsp. coconut sugar

* Blend mylk, pineapple and sugar in a blender
* Pour into glass jars
* Stir in chia seeds
* Leave 20 or more minutes
* Eat

- - ♥ - -

MANGO CHIA PUDDING

1 cup coconut mylk or other nut mylk
½ cup chopped mango
2 tbsp. chia seeds
2 tbsp. maple syrup or 1 tbsp. coconut sugar

* Blend mylk, mango and sugar in a blender
* Pour into glass jars
* Stir in chia seeds
* Leave 20 or more minutes
* Eat

JAM CHIA PUDDING
1 cup coconut mylk or other nut mylk
2-3 tbsp. fruit jam
2 tbsp. chia seeds
few drops or ½ tsp. vanilla
2 tbsp. maple syrup or 1 tbsp. coconut sugar

* Stir in glass jar
* Place in fridge
* Leave 20 or more minutes
* Eat

Tip: Read ingredients of jam. Only buy jam with fruit as the first ingredient which means it is the main ingredient. Jams with sugar as the first ingredient mean they have more sugar than fruit in the jar.

- - ♡ - -

CHIA FRUIT ON TOP PARFAITS
1 cup vanilla or chocolate
already made chia pudding

* Fill glass with chia pudding
* Top with fruit, fruit puree, jam, cacao nibs, nuts or seeds
* Eat

PETRA'S FAVORITE CHIA PUDDING

1 cup coconut mylk (fresh or the cream can kind)

1 tbsp. raw cacao powder

1 tbsp. coconut sugar

2 tbsp. chia seeds

* Blend mylk, cacao and sugar in a blender
* Pour into glass jars
* Stir in chia seeds
* Place in fridge
* Leave 20 or more minutes
* Eat

- - ♥ - -

PETRA'S FAVORITE CHIA SNACK

* Chop watermelon
* Place in bowl
* Add chocolate chia pudding on top
* Eat - YUM!!!

- - ♥ - -

PETRA'S 2ND FAVORITE CHIA SNACK

* Chop watermelon, pineapple, papaya in small cubes
* Place in bowl
* Add chocolate chia pudding on top
* Eat - YUM!!!

CHIA LAYERED PARFAITS

* Fill 1/3 glass with chia pudding
* Add a layer of fruit, fruit puree, jam, cacao nibs, nuts, seeds, raisins, goji berries or shredded coconut
* Fill 2/3 glass with more chia pudding
* Add a layer of fruit, fruit puree, jam, cacao nibs, nuts, seeds, raisins, goji berries or shredded coconut
* Fill 3/3 with more chia pudding
* Top with fruit, fruit puree, jam, cacao nibs, nuts, seeds, raisins, goji berries or shredded coconut
* Eat

- - ♡ - -

CHAPTER 41

LET'S MAKE
ICE CREAM

H ERE IS A SIMPLE YUMMY ICE CREAM DESSERT
that I can make to transition me into my JUICY cleanse
and also have as part of my future JUICY lifestyle. There
are many vegan JUICY ice cream recipes I can explore using
nut mylks as my base and this recipe is even simpler than that.

I blend frozen fruit with a little coconut water or
coconut mylk in a blender to make a frosty smoothie ice cream
bowl. I can add fruit and cacao nibs on top and I have the most
delicious sweet JUICY snack.

The best fruit for this ice cream are frozen bananas and
they make the perfect base to add other fruit flavors to. Frozen
mango, blueberries, papaya and dragon fruit also make a great
ice cream base as they all blend up smooth and creamy.

JUICY BANANA ICE CREAM

2 cups frozen banana chunks
$^3/_4$ cup coconut mylk, nut mylk or coconut water

Add Superfoods: Raw cacao, maca, lacuma, hemp seeds, chia
seeds, coconut oil, shredded coconut, chopped nuts,
chopped seeds on top or into the banana mixture

- - ♡ - -

JUICY FRUITY ICE CREAM

2 cups frozen fruit chunks
$^3/_4$ cup coconut mylk, nut mylk or coconut water

Add Superfoods: Raw cacao, maca, lacuma, hemp seeds, chia
seeds, coconut oil, shredded coconut, chopped nuts,
chopped seeds on top or into the fruit mixture

Best Frozen Fruit: Bananas, Dragon Fruit, Mango,
Blueberries, Papaya

2nd Best Frozen Fruit: Pineapple, Raspberries, Strawberries,

- - ♡ - -

CHAPTER 42

LET'S MAKE TEA

TEA IS VERY MEDICINAL AND HEALING FOR my body. The type of tea and the quality of ingredients is super important. Black tea is not as healthy for me as it is mainly caffeine and teeth staining. Herbal teas can soothe my digestive track, heal my illnesses, balance my hormones, lower my blood pressure, activate my brain, ease pain in my body, relax my muscles, boost my immune system and heal cancer. The list goes on and on. I buy good quality loose leaf teas that are ideally organic and non radiated. This is medicine so I make sure to get a good quality kind.

The rule with tea making is...

Loose leaf teas get added to already boiled / hot water and left to steep to extract their medicines. They are not boiled.

Root teas get boiled and then simmered to extract their medicines.

VARIOUS CLEANSING LOOSE LEAF TEAS...

Nettle
Green tea
Dandelion leaf
Moringa
Mate
Passion Flower
Other mixes

VARIOUS CLEANSING ROOT TEAS...

Ginger
Turmeric
Astragalas

VARIOUS CLEANSING MUSHROOM TEAS...

Chaga
Reishi

Chaga is a super medicinal mushroom used in Chinese medicine for centuries. It is used to reduce tumors, boost the immune system and rebuild my body on a cellular level. It grows like a black charcoal fungus on birch trees and can only be removed with an ax. It has a delicious coffee like similarity that when coconut mylk is added, it can give me that same coffee creamy feeling. It is also delicious blended with few tea spoons of coconut sugar and few tea spoons of coconut oil in a blender to make a delicious latee. Or I can drink it black. If I drink coffee, then during my JUICY lifestyle I can add chaga tea to coffee to super hero level up my coffee.

PETRA'S FAVORITE CHAGA TEA

1 chunk of chaga mushroom or few teaspoons chaga powder
4 cups spring water

* Soak chaga in water overnight
* Bring water to almost boil
* Simmer for 20 minutes
* Drink tea black
* Or add coconut milk and sweetener for coffee like taste

- - ♡ - -

PETRA'S FAVORITE CHAGA LATTE

1 cup hot already made chaga tea
2 tsp. coconut oil
2 tsp. coconut sugar

* Place all ingredients into a blender
* Blend
* Coconut oil will turn into a lattee
* Enjoy
* Alternate Option: ½ cup coffee and ½ cup chaga tea

- - ♡ - -

PETRA'S MAUI JUNGLE SUPER TEA

1 finger grated ginger root
2 fingers grated turmeric root
4 cups spring water

Optional: cardamom or lemon grass

* Place all ingredients in a pot
* Lightly boil for 5 minutes
* Drink tea

* When tea finished add 4 more cups water to used roots
* Boil for 10 minutes
* When tea finished add 4 more cups water to used roots
* Boil for 15 minutes

This tea can be boiled a few times always increasing the boil time to get the last bits of medicine out. I can add coconut mylk to make this tea creamy and more filling for my JUICY cleanse. I can have a pot of this tea on the stove at all times, always adding more water. When I have tea ready, I ensure I will drink it.

- - ♥ - -

CHAPTER 43

LET'S TALK BREAD

I KNOW EVERYONE LOVES BREAD!!! Most likely, I love it too! I might not feel that good after eating wheat gluten bread or I might not even notice the effect of gluten on my system until I take it out. Maybe without even realizing it, bread makes me feel bloated and puffy. I can now try switching wheat bread, crackers, pasta to organic rice and corn brands instead.

I might love croissants or other wheat pastries that don't have gluten free options. That is ok. I can eat wheat croissants on occasion and give myself permission to do so. If I bless up my food and put the intention in that it will be good for my body, then my body will be better equipped to handle the allergens.

Gluten is a natural allergen to my body. Some people are noticeably allergic to gluten and have Celiac disease. Celiac disease is an auto immune reaction to eating gluten where the small intestine can not handle this allergen. Most likely all of us are allergic to gluten in some form. When I cut this one allergen out of my diet, I will see how quickly my health and energy improves.

Eating gluten makes me tired, sluggish, activates my allergies, causes inflammation in my body, is a leading cause of arthritis or joint pain and is tough on my digestive system. Gluten can also make me fat and puffy. I might not notice the effects of gluten in my body until I remove it for a few weeks and then introduce it back in.

If I am eating some food during my JUICY food cleanse, then I at least stop eating gluten to give my body a break from this allergen. As I move into my JUICY lifestyle, I will continue removing gluten out of my diet completely.

Most likely gluten gives me a stuffy nose, bloats my stomach and makes me way more tired. Gluten is causing inflammation inside my body and is causing my small intestine and gut to flare up due to the irritation it is experiencing. Inflammation is at the cause of most sickness and is also at the stem of joint pain, arthritis and most body aches.

Most people feel tired after eating gluten because the body has to work extra hard to process this allergen and it takes all of the body's energy for digestion. For my JUICY lifestyle, I switch my wheat products for GLUTEN FREE alternatives like rice, corn, quinoa and buckwheat. I will not be missing anything, just making healthier choices.

Another huge thing is that conventional wheat is sprayed with Glyphosate (Monsanto's Weed Killer - Round Up), which is a pesticide that causes much harm. It is sprayed on conventional wheat to expedite the drying process, so the grain can get to the market faster and make the farmer more $$$. But it is super toxic and is sprayed on conventional wheat, oats, rice and edible beans.

Glyphosate causes nutritional deficiencies, especially minerals and systemic toxicity. It causes multiple chronic diseases and ruins my gut bacteria which then affects my entire system. It affects my hormone system and creates an imbalance. Traces of it are found in unborn fetuses and it causes many birth defects. Most people with chronic illnesses have high doses of glyphosate in their blood stream. The corporations will say it washes off the food and is not harmful for us, but natural doctors would disagree when seeing the harmful health effects from this WEED KILLER swimming in our blood stream. High traces of glyphosate is the common cause of Hodgkin's lymphoma cancer and other cancers plaguing people today.

Cleansing will help me remove this toxin out of my body. Starting a JUICY lifestyle and removing gluten out of my diet will help me eliminate glyphosate out of my food supply. If I choose to eat wheat and gluten, I then buy organic to avoid glyphosate.

FEW WAYS TO SWITCH GLUTEN OUT OF MY DIET...

These are for my JUICY lifestyle AFTER my JUICY cleanse.

1. GLUTEN FREE RICE PASTA - Tinkyada is a great store bought brand. Tastes the same but does not bloat me up. I will have a lot more energy after eating a big bowl of rice pasta instead feeling my energy drop when I eat a big bowl of wheat pasta.

2. GLUTEN FREE CEREALS – Usually made from puffed rice, corn or quinoa. There are many varieties and flavors. I will love the energy and good feeling I have after eating a bowl of gluten free cereal with fresh fruit and my homemade almond mylk. I always read ingredients, as even the organic brands can have unnecessary fillers like soy and use toxic canola oil. I avoid these brands.

3. GLUTEN FREE BREAD – There are a few rice breads, quinoa and nut breads that are delicious. Most gluten free bread is more firm, dry and dense than regular fluffy white bread. Usually found in the freezer section of healthy grocer stores as they do not contain preservatives. It tastes the best when toasted and yummy spreads are applied. I try spreading almond butter, cashew cream cheeses and healthy jams on my new gluten free toast as part of my new JUICY lifestyle.

4. GLUTEN FREE WRAPS – I now switch from eating wheat wraps to non-gmo corn tortillas that are made pure (corn, salt, lime & water) or quinoa or rice paper wraps. I read the ingredients of everything I buy, even if it says organic. Corn tortillas are an awesome staple food to have on hand for my JUICY lifestyle. I can wrap up anything and make quick food. I can wrap up my salads, veggies, beans, rice and stew dishes. Corn tortillas need to be heated on a pan before being eaten to soften them. They taste delicious and I won't be able to eat just one.

5. GLUTEN FREE RICE CRACKERS – Lots of flavors and varieties. Easy to get hooked on this new snack and never miss wheat crackers again.

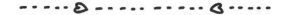

GLUTEN MAKES ME TIRED & SLUGGISH
IRRATATES MY BELLY
CAUSES INFLAMMATION IN MY BODY
AND MAKES ME PUFFY
I LET GO OF GLUTEN NOW
I LOVE MYSELF
I FEED MYSELF HEALING FOOD

- - ♡ - -

CHAPTER 44

LET'S TALK DAIRY

W E ARE THE ONLY MAMMALS ON THE PLANET that still drink milk into adult hood. The only reason I am drinking cows milk instead of gorilla milk, for example, is because cows are easier to heard, abuse and produce much more milk. Gorillas would not put up with much abuse and would get angry pretty fast. The rest of society and I could also be drinking dog milk, cat milk or pig milk if we were programmed long enough. Yuck!

I have been brainwashed to believe that certain food is good for me when it is not. I've been programmed to drink milk, lots of it and believe it is good for me and for my bones. The food pyramid I grew up on was funded by the meat, dairy and egg industry. My teachers and the government told me it was good for me and I obeyed without questioning, until now.

Unlike the old days, milk is now pasteurized which changes the chemical make up of the food and kills all the enzymes that are needed for my easy digestion. If a new born cow was fed pasteurized milk instead of raw milk, it would die within a few days. Pasteurized milk has no life sustaining and thriving value since the nutrients are pasteurized and killed.

If I am not a vegan yet and I still consume dairy products, then eating unpasteurized raw sheep, goat or cow dairy is much healthier for me. Raw is the only way I should consume dairy products. Raw dairy is full of enzymes that my body understands and can digest. Raw dairy can be used as medicine to heal major gut sicknesses and immune problems. If I need this level of healing, then ideally I would buy my own sheep, goat or cow and treat this animal with total love and respect for the purpose of my healing. I can also buy raw milk from certain "beat the system" local farmers that are treating their animals with care. If I need this as medicine, I can expedite healing my immune system, other gut and body sicknesses with this modality.

Sometimes people's bodies can get quite messed up by the medical industry, pharmaceutical drugs and really poor eating habits, that using raw animal products is the only way they can heal. It is not for everyone, especially if I am a vegan, but for some people survival is their only goal. Many people with severe stomach and immune issues, need help from the animal kingdom for their healing. There are many families that end up buying a sheep or goat to feed their children raw milk. A lot of neurological and immune diseases have been helped by raw dairy, when the person felt like they had no more options left. In most places raw dairy is illegal, which is ridiculous because that is how our ancestors ate. I can get raw dairy from certain farms if I purchase a share of the cow. Most raw dairy places are watched extra closely by the FDA and government regulations that don't like alternative medicine accessible to the people. I can take my health into my hands and choose what is right for me. No one has this power over me.

Vegetarian, Vegan, Cruelty Free and Raw Food lifestyles are journeys I embark on to awaken my consciousness, heal my body to the next level and take care to heal the planet.

As part of my JUICY lifestyle, becoming a vegan or vegetarian means I am eating lots of raw food, raw greens and good fats as part of my diet plan. There are many vegans and vegetarians who don't eat vegetables. Eating a diet of mainly potato chips, donuts and processed food could label me as a vegan or a vegetarian, but it does not mean I am eating healthy. Becoming a vegan means compassion for animals, compassion for the environment and compassion for myself. Eating the most amazing JUICY life force food is an incredible way I LOVE myself.

My body is naturally allergic to dairy and I lack the digestive enzymes needed for digestion. In the past popping lactose pills, suffering with bloating and stomach cramps was all worth it for a big bowl of ice cream but now, with so many dairy alternatives, I do not have to suffer any more and I don't need to eat milk to enjoy ice cream. I also don't need to bother animals to get my cold icey treat.

Removing dairy out of my JUICY lifestyle will give me LOTS OF BENEFITS and I will do good for the animals, the planet and feel so much better in my body. I might not realize that I am allergic to dairy. When I eat something for so long, I might not be able to tell how it is affecting me until I remove it and see how much better I feel.

Dairy is an allergen and causes acidity in my body. Acidity causes my body to be on fire and creates inflammation. Inflammation is at the root of most sickness. When my body is on fire, it has a harder time of self healing. Dairy also causes my body to produce excess mucous, as a way of expelling the toxin. So when I eat dairy, I add extra phlegm into my body. Little kids, who are over exposed to dairy, have snotty noses and ear infections because their body is trying to push out the excess toxic dairy mucous.

Conventional milk is full of antibiotics and hormones that are pumped into the cow. Cows are fed genetically modified hormone altering corn and this crap goes into the milk also. The FDA and governments keep raising the amount of pus allowed in milk, so each carton of milk is full of pus from the sore teats of cows being milked way too often. Cows are over milked for mass production to make the most amount of $$$ and their teats are sore, bleeding and pussing right into my conventional milk, cheese and yogurt products.

I start making my own nut mylks for my coffee, cereals and smoothies. A can of Thai coconut milk is my new dairy switch staple and is perfect for coffees, soups, curries and smoothies. I can dilute 1 can of coconut milk to 2 cans of water to make my own super quick dairy free nut mylk.

Cheese is addictive and the casein, is the addictive element. Casein found in cheese is more closely linked to cancer, than smoking is linked to breast cancer. This might shock me enough to stop eating cheese forever.

Bye, bye dairy and bye, bye cheese! This is my JUICY lifestyle and I am worth it. If I am not ready to release dairy yet, then I release it during my JUICY cleanse to give my body a digestive break.

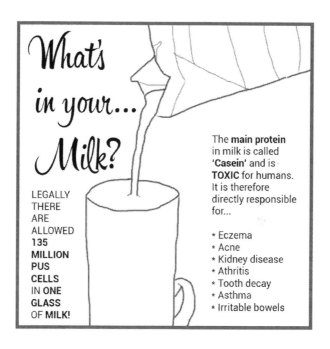

What's in your... Milk?

LEGALLY THERE ARE ALLOWED **135 MILLION PUS CELLS** IN **ONE GLASS** OF **MILK!**

The **main protein** in milk is called **'Casein'** and is **TOXIC** for humans. It is therefore directly responsible for...

* Eczema
* Acne
* Kidney disease
* Athritis
* Tooth decay
* Asthma
* Irritable bowels

I also remember that a cow, sheep or goat do not just naturally carry milk around. Animals are the same as humans and only produce milk because they had a baby. So if I drink dairy or eat cheese, I am sharing milk that is meant for the baby. On conscious family farms, baby cows get the milk and all extra is taken for human consumption. Happy well taken care of grass fed cows continue producing milk naturally. In the conventional mass dairy industry momma cows are stripped away from their babies instantly and put into milking troughs. They cry and scream for their babies but no one listens or cares. This sadness and terror energy goes into every carton of milk and package of cheese I buy. Food is energy and the dairy, egg and meat industry has a lot of torture and pain energy in the products I buy.

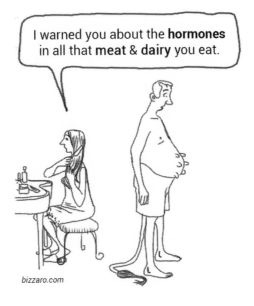

VEGAN NO DAIRY CHEESE RECIPES...

ALMOND VEGAN BAKED CHEESE
1.5 cups almond meal
1/4 cup lemon juice
1/4 cup water
3 tbsp. olive oil
1 clove garlic
1/2 tsp. pink salt

* Blend all together in food processor
* Stir in additional herbs or various flavor combinations
* Pour into bake dish or mould into round cheese on bake tray
* Bake for 180 Celcius for 25 min

- - ♥ - -

RAW CASHEW CREAMY CHEESE
1.5 cup soaked cashews (2 hrs or overnight)
3 tbsp. nutritional yeast
2 tbsp. fresh lemon juice
1/4 tsp. garlic powder
1/2 tsp. pink salt
1/4 tsp. black pepper
1/4 cup spring water

* Rinse soaked cashews and throw out the water
* Blend cashews and spring water in food processor
* Blend in rest of ingredients and season to taste

A LOVE NOTE FROM PETRA: When I first got into the health movement I became PLANT BASED with some raw dairy, rooster fertilized farm fresh eggs and raw cheese. I joined a raw dairy co-op in Vancouver and owned ¼ share of a cow. My money paid for the care of this animal and I had access to raw yogurt, milk, cheese and butter delivered to me by the farmer. I knew the farm was ethical and I loved that they were STANDING UP to the SYSTEM that prevents us-humans from milking our own cows and sharing that milk with others out of our FREE WILL and SOVEREIGNTY, as our BIRTH RIGHT on this planet. I really believe in all of us stepping into our sovereignty as humans on this planet, as we are the ones that are allowing our enslavement, when we do not speak up for our free rights. SO SPEAK UP!!!

More and more, I moved away from eating animal products as I more and more, believed in the SOVEREIGNTY of animals on this planet TOO. So I let go of raw dairy and raw cheeses as I no longer want to contribute to the mass cruelty, torture, slaughter and biggest injustice we have on this planet the MEAT, DAIRY and EGG industry. Even if it is ethical, I now question if I need to bother an animal to eat abundantly and like a queen. If I focus on my raw plant based path, then I definitely do not and can make the MOST AMAZING raw cheeses and creamy spreads plant based style!

CHAPTER 45

LET'S TALK MEAT

D URING MY JUICY CLEANSE, I CUT OUT MEAT to give my body a digestive break. For my new JUICY lifestyle, I move towards eating LESS meat or cutting it out forever. This JUICY cleanse will help me flush out old waste living inside my system. Most likely this old waste is undigested meat and excess fecal matter.

If I continue being a meat eater, then it is essential I drink green smoothies, juices, liquids and eat more raw food to flush myself out every day. I don't want undigested rotting meat chunks living inside my body slowly causing me harm. Ideally I let go of eating red meat and pork as fast as possible as these two meats will cause the most amount of harm to my health. Then I eventually let go of chicken, lamb, turkey and fish too. Fish is full of mercury, micro plastics and toxic harmful chemicals making it no longer a healthier alternative meat option. I definitely stay away from farmed salmon and always ask if it is farmed or wild before buying.

I allow my EATING and BUYING choices to create less animal slaughter and torture on this planet. Beef is the worst contaminating and environment deteriorating industry on this planet. It is the biggest contributor to global warming and robs most of the planet's fresh water supply to produce beef. Beef is the worst for my body to digest. It takes over 12 hours to digest a piece of steak in my body. It seems crazy when I imagine my system trying to digest a giant steak. My teeth can't rip it so I need a big sharp steak knife to break it apart. If my teeth can't rip it, then I start to wonder if my body is really designed to eat meat.

For more health, awareness and empowerment, I watch these films.
1. Forks Over Knives
2. Cowspiracy
3. Earthlings

PERHAPS I MAKE THIS STATEMENT NOW...

"For my health, the health of the planet and the survival of humanity, I now bother animals less and less for my daily food supply and lifestyle choices. I slowly cut out meat, dairy, cheese and eggs. I stop buying all animal hide products like leather shoes, bags, key chains, wallets, jackets, goose down feathers and real fur stuff too. I love and honor any animal products I do have, and am grateful to the animal that lost its life so I can carry a fancy purse around. I am now awake, aware and more conscious of how I spend my money."

If I am already a vegan, I move towards a more raw fresh food lifestyle and limit my intake of vegan fake soy meat, white bread, white sugar, donuts and French fries. Just because it is on a vegan menu, doesn't mean it is healthy. Soy is an allergen to my body. Saitan is made from gluten, which is another allergen to my body. White sugar and white flour, which most vegan desserts are made from, are death for my body. So I read ingredients and remember it is for the compassion of animals, for the compassion of the planet and for the compassion of MYSELF that I am a vegan.

I celebrate me! I am proud for making this profound diet and lifestyle choice. I am proud for stepping outside the box, being a leader and showing others a better way to eat and live.

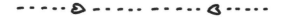

A LOVE NOTE FROM PETRA: I started letting go of meat when I was researching ways to heal my mom naturally of cancer. I learned how toxic meat is for our body and how it, along with dairy and cheese, are the foods that cause us cancer. Since not getting cancer was my goal after my mom passed away, I let go of this poison and started teaching others to do the same. I first let go of beef, pork and all shellfish as they are the most toxic for our body. I then let go of chicken and turkey. After a while I also let go of fish.

Eating is an evolution and a journey. I invite you to see it that way and evolve as a super human on this planet using food as your medium. I no longer eat any animal flesh. I grew up eating killed back yard rabbits and chickens. I nibbled on cooked pig tails and chicken necks with my dad as a normal eating ritual. I cracked open bones to suck the marrow out of them. My family ate the whole animal and we were connected to our meat as I grew up. As my eating journey continued and I cleansed my body on many levels, I moved into plant based and eat mainly raw for ultimate health.

During my period time, my body always craves something "EXTRA" and I used to give myself fish during these few days when I felt really out of balance. Having given up flesh, I now eat an egg from time to time, as this is sometimes the only way I feel I can balance. I make sure to only eat eggs from a local farmer who is treating his chickens with love. I am constantly moving away from eating eggs and am finding alternative sources of protein for my body. I eat lots of kale, lentils, chia seeds, hemp seeds, hummus and coconut yogurt. I experiment with increasing more good fats, plant proteins and good salts into my diet and move away from my conditioned, since I was a child, body desire for animal fat and animal protein.

I don't believe most of us crave meat as much as we crave the fat and salt. Most new vegetarians say that bacon is the hardest to give up. Why? Because it is fat that our body craves not the flesh of another sentient species. So I invite you to explore adding more good fats into your diet and see how much your body cravings change and how much better your body feels.

I also no longer contribute to the animal industry, via buying leather shoes, bags, Uggs, sheep skins, animal tested cosmetics or any products made from animal skin. I will not throw out what I already have.

I honor the animal that died for my shoes, the sheep that got skinned for my sheep skin rugs and the ducks that were live plucked for my goose jacket and duvets. When I purchased these items, I was asleep to the reality of this cruel industry and disconnected to the lives of the animals I was wearing. So I choose to no longer contribute to the cruelty and suffering of innocent animals, tortured for us humans on this planet and I vote with my dollars. Please do the same. Your life is worth it. Love you, Petra

- - ♥ - -

CHAPTER 46

LET'S TALK SOY

I HAVE BEEN BRAINWASHED BY THE VEGETARIAN movement that soy, tofu and saitan are my healthy meat substitutes. I have been brainwashed that if I stop eating meat, that I should start eating soy for my protein.

Majority of the soy beans on the planet are owned by Monsanto, aka the devil. It is the only seed on the planet that is owned by a corporation. It is genetically modified (GMO) in a lab and I have no idea what these scientific and Frankenstein modifications will do to my body in the long run. Some countries, like Australia don't have GMO soy and many countries like Europe used to forbid Monsanto and GMO food to enter their countries, but now Monsanto and GMO food are all over Europe and all over the world. Monsanto has been in Asia since the 1970s and most Balinese rice is genetically modified along with the tofu everyone eats in mass quantities.

If I choose to eat tofu and soy, I research the brand to buy. Soy, tofu, tempe, saitan are not part of the JUICY lifestyle diet plan. They are acidic and increase the levels of harmful inflammation inside my body. Soy increases estrogen in my body effecting my hormone levels and is an allergen to my body causing me inflammation.

I research about all the healthy and the not so healthy benefits of soy, tempe and saitan and feel what resonates with me. If I chose to eat it, I eat it in moderation and eat more raw food and green smoothies. Ideally I eat fermented soy in the form of tempe or other fermented recipes, which make soy much healthier for my body. If I love it and I believe in it, then I enjoy it. But for the sake of my health and the health of the planet, I DON'T EAT GENETICALLY MODIFIED SOY.

G̟MO
FOODS TO AVOID

Cotton
Soy
Corn
Zucchini
Sugar
Papayas
Dairy
Apples
Canola
Yellow Squash

A LOVE NOTE FROM PETRA: I don't eat soy. I don't eat tofu. I don't touch soy milk. I don't eat saitan. I don't eat tempeh. I don't believe in it and I don't believe in the health benefits. Even if it is non GMO, I won't eat it. I like some tempeh if it is made from mung beans or alternative beans to soy. So as a general rule, I don't eat anything made from soy except edamame beans and I love those!

I don't eat the fake meats, soy, tofu or seitan based vegan food, I never have. I believe it is harmful for the body causing inflammation, which is at the cause of all sickness. As I released flesh meat from my diet, I didn't need to switch to fake meats because I was choosing super hero level health instead of trying to trick my mind to believe I am still eating meat food.

If you are letting go of meat and buying vegan "chicken" fingers or vegan hot dogs or tofu and it helps you transition, then GO FOR IT! I support you in letting go of meat, which is much worse for your body health and the planet health. I invite you to release the soy processed food when you are ready, knowing there is even a healthier way to eat. SUPER HERO style!

- - ♡ - -

I DO THIS CLEANSE FOR ME

I TAKE THIS TIME FOR ME

I HEAL MY BODY FOR ME

I LOVE ME

I TAKE CARE OF ME

I AM WORTH IT

- - ♡ - -

CHAPTER 47

LET'S TALK SUGAR

T HIS NASTY LITTLE KILLER, also known as WHITE DEATH, is slowly poisoning the minds and bodies of people everywhere, including perhaps me. White sugar stops my immune system from working for over 20 minutes. Just stops it. No more immune system. Shuts down for over 20 minutes.

Now imagine that as a mom I feed my kids candy or sugary cereals or processed food with tons of sugar added in and wonder why my children get sick. Or it is I who eats sugary cereals, cakes, cookies and candy full of white death and wonder why I don't feel or look that great. Or imagine that while I am in the hospital trying to heal, they feed me jello, soft drinks, candies and ice cream full of immune suppressing sugar. Or imagine I stay home from work sick and eat a box of sugar filled chocolate to feel better. Instead of healing myself with raw chocolate, I have just lowered my immune system and my ability to heal.

Sugar is like crack cocaine and we, including me, are all legally addicted to it. Have I ever tried to take Halloween candy away from a child or tried to part with my last piece of cake or donut? It is quite scary to witness.

Sugar contributes to most of my health problems, obesity issues, improperly functioning organs and is the root cause of my potential dis-ease. So I cut the white crap out and become healthy again. Time to remove this white death out of my life forever before it creates more and more harm.

As part of my JUICY cleanse, I cut out white sugar and all processed sugars to give my digestive system a break. As part of my JUICY lifestyle, I cut out white sugar and switch to coconut sugar, maple syrup and stevia. I start reading the ingredients of everything I buy, as sugar sneaks into so much packaged food and has many names. Two of the nastiest I avoid are HIGH FRUCTOSE CORN SYRUP and ASPARTAME aka Equal, NutraSweet and NatraTaste Blue. More artificial harmful sweeteners I avoid are Sucralose (Splenda), Acesulfame K (Ace k, Sunette, Equal Spoonful, Sweet One, Sweet 'n Safe), Saccharin (Sweet N Low, Sweet Twin), Xylitol and Sorbitol. They are all very toxic and harmful to my health, neurological system and they make me fat.

I cut sugary foods and drinks out of my diet, as much as possible, and stop adding teaspoons of sugar to all my drinks. I know it is addictive and it can be hard for me to let this one go, but I have to if I want to be thriving on this planet. I can still have sweet desserts and yummy delicious food, I just make sure it is made with real sugar or dates or fruit sugar, rather than the white chemical crap. Once I release white sugar and sugary things out of my diet, I will notice my body craves it less and less. Once my taste buds cleanse, I will not crave sugar so much.

For my JUICY lifestyle, the easiest solution to my sugar cravings is to switch to making or buying raw vegan desserts and raw cacao chocolate. Raw vegan desserts are chemical free, white sugar free, gluten free, wheat free, soy free, dairy free and food coloring free. They are natural whole food made from nuts, fruits, seeds, cacao and natural sweeteners. I can eat cake sin free for breakfast, lunch or dinner. I can also eat boxes and boxes of raw chocolates and never feel guilty again. Chocolate, in its natural form, is really healthy and healing for me. It is when white sugar, soy, dairy and other crap is added to the chocolate that it becomes unhealthy.

Raw chocolate is full of magnesium which is needed for me to thrive in my health and it also helps oxygenate my colon so I poo better. Magnesium is considered the spark of life in my body and needed for all my joints, nerves and organs to function properly. I stop producing magnesium after I turn 30 years and need to supplement it to thrive. It is the salt found in the ocean and in natural Epsom salts, which I absorb via my skin when I soak in the salty water. I can also add magnesium to my body with a magnesium water spray and I can EAT LOTS OF RAW CHOCOLATE. When I crave chocolate it is my body actually craving magnesium and so I eat LOTS totally guilt free. If I have a sweet tooth then I don't deny myself, I just eat sweets that will be healing for my body instead of harmful.

I LOOK IN THE MIRROR
I LOVE WHO IS LOOKING BACK
I WINK AND WAVE AT MYSELF
I LOVE MYSELF
I AM PROUD OF MYSELF
I AM HAPPY TO BE ME

- - ♡ - -

CHAPTER 48

LET'S TALK WEIGHT LOSS

I F I DON'T FEEL MY IDEAL WEIGHT, THEN I DO something about it. If I don't feel good in my skin body bag and it is not much fun cruising around the world in my body spaceship, then I make a change. Only I can choose to make this change, and this JUICY cleanse and JUICY lifestyle WILL HELP ME!

Sometimes I just do the same thing over and over because I don't know any different. I was never taught to eat healthy and most likely my parents didn't know either. I never knew about cleansing my system to run optimally. This book has now taught me to open my mind, teach me that I can eat differently and I can actually heal my body. I can finally start loving the body I am in and feel good physically every day. Maybe my JUICY cleanse will not get rid of all my discomforts at once, but it is a great start to my healthier life. My JUICY cleanse will help me lose weight, have more energy and feel happier in my body so I jump out of bed in the morning inspired for my new life.

So why am I overweight? I ask myself this question and allow my intuition to answer. Maybe I know the answer right away or maybe I have to dig a little deep. Is the extra weight to protect me and keep me safe in some way? Is it as a result of fear, insecurities and not wanting to be the greatest version of myself for some reason? Is it that I just don't love my body or myself enough, no matter what weight I am?

Why do I want to lose weight? What will a skinnier, healthier body do for me? I close my eyes and see my new healthier skinnier body. How do I feel? How is my life different in a body that I feel good in?

Issues live in the tissues and some unresolved emotional issue is most likely why I am overweight. Energetically extra weight is extra padding, extra protection and more safety within my body spaceship. It can be a form of hiding from the opposite sex or from myself. It can be a physical representation of all the self loathing, sadness and insecurity I have inside. It can be a way to hide who I truly am and who I am too afraid to express.

Excess weight is a form of self punishment and self loathing. I cannot adore my body and all its organs and feed them poison at the same time. Excess weight is also a lot of preasure on all my organs so they don't feel loved. When I have excess weight, I am not connected to my body and how it functions. I am not connected to choosing food as my fuel or my poison. Perhaps I don't realize that most sickness is a lifestyle eating disease which I can prevent and heal with my JUICY cleanse and with simple switches to my more JUICY lifestyle. Maybe I don't realize I have the power and the self worth to have a body vessel I feel really good in. Maybe I don't feel I deserve to feel good, to be really happy or to love myself. Well it is time to change all that.

Cleansing physically with juices, smoothies and raw food will help flush out my toxins, release the excess weight and the excess crap I have been carrying around and as I flush my body, I have to flush my mind too. I start flushing down the toilet the old disempowering, critical, judgmental, self loathing, self diminishing and small minded thinking. I flush down shame, guilt, not enoughness, fear and the scarcity mind set I have been carrying around. It is time to purge my mind and start loving myself if I want to get rid of my weight and have it stay off.

When I adore my body and myself so much that I only feed myself JUICY healthy vibrant food and think only JUICY healthy vibrant thoughts, then I will naturally lose the weight. My body is waiting for me to love it, to become best friends with it and to start working together for my greatest thrival on this planet. It's time to start connecting to myself, loving my body and healing my heart.

As I start JUICY cleansing, my emotions, hurts and wounds will float up to the surface. I will feel them and they will feel crappy. Everything in me will want to eat a giant pasta meal, a donut, a cookie or a big greasy sandwich to stuff these emotions back down. I DON'T DO IT!!! I don't push the old crap back down to rot for many more years, I get rid of it now forever.

How do I get rid of my emotions, wounds, hurts, regrets, shames and pains forever? I go for it and I do this JUICY cleanse and give my body time for healing. When my emotions and pains start to surface and I want to explode, I feel them. I have to feel them, to heal them. I keep feeling them and I say, "thank you, I love you, I forgive you and I let you go". As I feel it and forgive things, I slowly heal them inside me. Old pain inside my body will cause me harm so I get it out. It might not be easy and I can do it. I am powerful, I am strong and I am worth it.

How do I do my JUICY cleanse so I lose more weight? I drink only liquids and lots of juices for 7 or more days. I give my body a break from digesting and I give it time for healing. I drink lots of healing liquids to keep flushing my crap out. I drink sweet or savory green smoothies every morning to scrape out my intestines. I do enemas and colonics to get the crap out fast. I clean my mouth every morning. I go to saunas and sweat my toxins out. I move my body. I love my body. I do mirror work and tell myself that I love myself. I become my own best friend and LOVE MYSELF! I become equanimities in my mind and I release all judgment and nasty inner self talk.

I am a whole energetic being. I let go of the physical as I let go of the mental. I heal as a whole being. I love myself and I am worth it.

CHAPTER 49

LET'S TALK GUT ISSUES

I F I HAVE GUT ISSUES THEN I WILL WANT TO do this JUICY cleanse as soon as possible. I might be suffering from some sort of bloating, constipation, cramping, farting, inflammation, heart burn, gout, Chrons, IBS or Colitis. It will be important for me to gauge how I heal myself and what kind of JUICY cleanse I embark on. If my conditions are quite sever, then green juice or green smoothies might be too intense at first on my inflamed raw guts.

This chapter only briefly touches on healing my gut. A more detailed conversation and online coaching with Petra is required to fully address all my gut issues and how to heal them.

Most of us have some form of gut issues. Our diet, our environment and our stress have contributed to our gut health being out of balance and us not feeling very well. Our gut might cause slight daily discomfort or it can keep us from being social as we always need a nearby toilet. What ever my issues are, I resolve them so I can live a happy, healthy and free life.

When I have gut issues, my digestive track and gut is inflamed and my gut flora is out of balance. My body should have more good gut bacteria than bad, but most likely I have an overgrowth of bad bacteria in my system. This bad bacteria causes candida, yeast infections, skin issues, weak hair, problem skin and creates an imbalance in my entire body system. The gut is the Queen to my system so if it is not happy, it shows up everywhere in my body.

This JUICY cleanse will help me. I start with stopping the intake of food that is hard to digest and possibly causing me harm. Flushing my system with JUICY liquids will heal my inflamed digestive track. Depending on how damaged my gut and digestive track are, a green juice might feel too strong and hurt my stomach. I will have to gauge what works for me and what doesn't. Perhaps drinking herbal stomach healing teas all day will do the trick. Perhaps a green smoothie will be okay but if my body is extremely damaged maybe bone broth soup is what will heal me. Sometimes bone broth soup is the only thing that can get my super damaged body back.

Bone broth is a bi product of the flesh eating industry and so many healing bones are discarded daily. Bones are actually the most alkaline part of the animal and the part that can help me with my gut healing. Meat is acidic and bones are alkaline. Meat eating animals chew and eat bones to alkaline their system. Ideally there is an end to the flesh eating industry and bone broth is no longer an option. It is likely that eating flesh and animal products is what hurt my gut in the first place. Yet if bones are available and I have severe gut inflammation issues, then bone broth soup might be my only source of help as it has helped many other sick people.

I try what works for me. I am gentle and love myself through this healing process. I first give my body a break from digesting so it can focus on my healing. If I want to eat food, then I eat simple food like quinoa, rice or potatoes that won't inflame my body any further. I eat gelatinous food like papaya, chia pudding, psyllium water and aloe vera to reduce the fire in my system. I eat a few tea spoons of coconut oil through out the day to cool and heal my digestive track.

I remember that stress is my biggest cause of digestive issues. So I STOP EATING STRESS. I use the power of my mind to remain calm, love myself and only treat myself with kindness and compassion. I only allow others to treat me the same. I create stronger boundaries and only do what feels good for me. I am in charge and this is my life. I love myself and take care of myself as number 1. I am worth it.

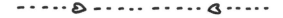

HOLDING ON TO RESENTMENT
IS LIKE DRINKING POISON
EXPECTING THE OTHER TO DIE

I FORGIVE MYSELF
I FORGIVE OTHERS
FOR ANY WRONG DOING

I AM WORTH THIS LEVEL OF HEALING

- - ♡ - -

CHAPTER 50

LET'S TALK ACHY BONES, JOINTS & PREMATURE AGING

EVERYONE WANTS TO LOOK YOUNGER AND HAVE a healthier body. Magazines are plastered with tips, tricks and products to reverse aging and most stars on our screens have frozen their faces with plastic surgery and Botox to maintain the forever young look. When I look in the mirror, perhaps I see all the extra weight, dark puffy circles and newly appearing wrinkles. As I get older, it may become harder to sit down and stand up, as my joints are stiffer and not as agile as before. Most likely I am living in a body that feels much older then I feel I am, but I don't know how to change that. I might have some form of arthritis, excess pudgy weight, old dull skin and achy bones.

It doesn't have to be this way. I can youthen my body, my face and physically feel I have reversed aging. I can have a flexible healthy moveable body once again.

I have got to do a JUICY cleanse. A cleanse to get rid of the toxins, the extra pudge, the excess fecal matter, clean my blood, alleviate my organs and have everything in my body working optimally again.

Most likely I am walking around dehydrated. I am not drinking enough liquids to cleanse my body and to nourish my thirsty cells. When my cells are thirsty and don't get enough liquid, they will start to dry up, shrivel and die. This type of cellular death is the leading cause of my premature aging. I am drying myself up and killing off my life force inside.

So JUICY cleansing is my answer. Time to spend 7+ days flushing my body with liquids and rehydrating all of my cells. My body will become JUICY once again and very HAPPY.

Most of my joint and body pain is a sign of inflammation inside my body. My body is on fire and it hurts. When I start drinking alkalizing cooling liquids, I will cool my body fire and take down my inflammation pain. At the stem of most sickness is inflammation, so by cleansing I stop the fire in its tracks. My arthritis and my joint pain will greatly reduce and ideally vanish. At the stem of arthritis is inflammation.

Without scaring myself too much, it is possible I have parasites inside my body that like to live in my joints. Parasites attack my immune system and weaken my entire body function. I am more susceptible to illness if my body is feeding parasites and they are excreting their poo into my body system. When I JUICY cleanse and flush out my body, I will help clean out all my joints and areas where parasites could be hiding. Drinking a teaspoon of food grade diatomaceous earth in water a few times per day throughout my cleanse will kill off my parasites. The diatomaceous earth is shards of glass on a microscopic level and it rips the bellies of these critters when they ingest it. When I flush out, I clean house. When I do my enemas and colonics, I take all my garbage out of my house and heal my body.

When I start drinking green and veggie juices, I will be filling my body with mass amount of nutrition and vitamins. My body is starving for this level of nutrition, which is also the cause of my aches and pains. When I nourish myself, I nourish every one of my cells, muscles, organs, tissues, and veins. All my aches and pains start to diminish as I lube up my body.

I think of my body like a car, I take care of it and it will run optimally for me. I neglect it and it will slowly start breaking down. If I am like a rusty deteriorating car, I start lubing myself up with the best car oil and fuel, so I can run optimally again.

I AM IN CHARGE OF
WHAT IS SAID IN MY HEAD
I CLOSE MY EYES
I LISTEN TO THE SELF TALK
I ONLY ALLOW KIND WORDS
I LET GO OF THE NASTY STUFF
MY MIND IS A TEMPLE
I ONLY ALLOW THE PURE IN

- - ♡ - -

CHAPTER 51

LET'S TALK CANCER

T HERE IS TOO MUCH INFORMATION TO WRITE in this small chapter to support me on my full cancer healing journey. Petra's coaching and online programs can help me further. In this chapter, I will get an introduction so I can start my cancer HEALING journey right now. Cancer is a journey into my own self and into my own healing.

Cancer is not the grim reaper coming to my door to collect me. NO! It is my own body knocking on my door saying, "HEY WAKE UP! What you are doing and how you are living is not working, so you have to change it or you will die faster than you want to. Let's make some changes and heal this body. Life isn't over for you yet." So I start listening to my body right now.

Cancer is not a monster that has attacked me, needs to be cut out, burned out or poisoned. Cancer is the co-creation between my mind, my heart, my soul, my body and the toxins I have inside. Usually it means that my body temple has gotten too toxic and can no longer self clean itself or function properly. Usually it means that I have lost myself and gotten disconnected from my heart. Usually it means that I am not listening to my soul's longings and my inner guidance system.

Cancer feeds on sugar and it feeds on stress. So I cut those out as fast as possible and CLEAN my body temple as fast as possible too. I do this JUICY cleanse right now! The faster I get the toxins out of my body, the faster my body can start to function again. Cancer cells have a broken on and off switch. As other cells in my body switch off and die as part of my body rhythm, cancer cells just stay turned on. Cleansing my body and nourishing it with green plant based liquids, repairs the cancer cell switch to turn off again. The cancer cells begin to die and new healthy cells grow in their place.

Doing a green JUICY cleanse and detox regime is imperative in healing my cancer naturally. Doing self love and forgiveness work is necessary for my healing too. I am a whole body being. I have to heal all of me for me to be healthy, happy and thriving.

I am very powerful and I can heal my cancer naturally. I start by getting rid of the toxins ingested by my mouth and by my mind. I don't let doctors scare me. I take my health into my hands. I do lots of research on natural healing. I get empowered and know I got this. I CAN heal my cancer naturally! I book a session with Petra or sign up for her online cancer healing program. I ask for help. I am worth it. My life is worth it.

EAT THIS DURING JUICY CANCER CLEANSING...

- lemon water
- wheat grass shots
- green juice
- carrot juice
- beet juice
- veggie juice
- savory green smoothie
- green raw soup
- coconut water
- alkaline water
- spring water
- charcoal water
- diatomaceous earth water
- bentonyte clay water
- spirulina water
- chlorella water
- chlorophyll water
- herbal teas
- essential oil water
- green salads and green veggies
- turmeric ginger shots

Food alone will not heal my cancer but it will be an amazing place to start. I then start focusing on waste removal, mindfulness, self love, forgiveness and mind perspective shifts. My healing will also involve healing toxic situations, toxic relationships, toxic events and toxic environments so my healing can happen on all levels. It will also involve letting go of old wounds, grief, guilt, shame and negative issues I am hanging on to.

Healing my cancer is a full on journey into my self if I am willing to go there. I will have to go into the dark places, the hidden places and the ugly places. I will have to go looking at things about myself that I don't want to look at, but I must look in order to heal. I must become my own best friend and completely adore myself so much. I must learn to love all the little parts of myself, even the icky parts. I have to choose to LIVE, no one can choose this for me. My family can be fighting for me to live and seeing me in my healing but if I am not convinced I will heal, then no healing will take place. No doctor, pill or therapy can heal me, only I can heal ME. Only I can choose to live, to heal and to get through this. I have to be willing to look at myself, to look at my life, to love myself and to learn from myself. I must get to know me. I must love to be me.

So if I have cancer, I strap on my seatbelt and go for the ride of my life in gratitude for this journey I am on. I have created cancer in my life so it's up to me to uncreate it. I wake up and make some changes in how I live my life. In the past, I might have been too afraid to make these changes or felt too lazy and this cancer is my wake up call. When I am faced with death, then my desire to live kicks in even stronger and I say f**ck this and I get myself healthy again.

I declared my end of victim consciousness in that moment and chose it to end for women everywhere. After 6 months and a biopsy scan, it was confirmed I was cancer free. I did lot of cleansing, belief changing and digging into the darkest parts of me, to transmute and heal.

I fully support your journey and I hope I have inspired you to know that cancer is NOT a death sentence but a knock on the door to change some things that have long needed changing!!!!

YOU ARE NOT ALONE! I GOT YOUR BACK! YOU GOT THIS!

I love you...Petra

CHAPTER 52

AFTER LOG & LOVE NOTE FROM PETRA

I sit here now, in Brno Czech republic writing the last chapters of this cleansing book. I am sharing an apartment in the city with my sweet daddy who is celebrating his 70th birthday and it is the purpose of this trip back to our birth land. He has many friends here and celebrates his birthday with ten other 70 year olds who he has known since he was 15 years old. So 150 people gathered in cabins in the woods and played guitar Czech tramp songs, drank keg Czech beer and ate lots of Czech style food. I flew from Bali. He flew from Canada. We met here in he Czech Republic.

Currently my dad is sick. He has a cold or a flu, fever,

sweats and excess phlegm. These are simple indicators that the body is trying to get rid of something. It is poisoned, over processed and needs to simplify. So it starts creating internal heat to push the toxins out of the skin. The body flushes the toxins out through the sweat and the mucous gets created to remove the crap out as well. It seems so simple for me to watch him. He arrived from Canada eating a pretty healthy diet. No gluten. No sugar. No processed food. Salads. Smoothies. Then arrives to the land of home made sausages, meats, cheeses, the most amazing cakes and desserts. Amazing home made pub food on every corner and the best yellow sweet potatoes on the planet. Slowly but steadily he goes for it. Sampling, snacking and enjoying food of his heritage.

His body can't handle it. A little cold air, a few cold drinks and his immune system can't hold back catching a cold.

Instead of cleansing the body and stopping all intake of allergens, as is the natural way, he is taking pharmaceutical pills to suppress the symptoms and get rid of his cold the pharmaceutical way.

Even though he is sharing the same living space with me, cleanse and detox expert, he is not ready for this way of healing. He believes in the doctor and fixing his cold the faster way, as the natural way is too radical for him. Cleansing, cleaning and stopping food he wants to eat, is not an option for him. So he can still eat food that is harming him and take pharmaceutical drugs to shut the body's messages down. The fever, the runny nose, the chills and the cough are all signals from the body telling us something is not working. It is only up to us if we choose to listen.

I bless everyone's journey and none of us can determine another's fate or how they should live their lives. Everyone is playing out their life movie and the only thing we can do is offer suggestions, knowledge and love without attachment to the outcome. My dad has chosen to go on antibiotics because he thinks this will heal his flu the fastest. He believes with his whole being, that this is the way you heal from sickness. If I would suggest that an enema could heal his fever and help his body rid itself of the toxins, he would freak out. He would say he is clean and that doing an enema has nothing to do with his healing.

Although he believes in conventional healing, I am happy that my dad is following some natural methods also. He is taking time to rest and lie down. He dresses warm and adds extra blankets on him, to help sweat his toxins out. He could however, take his sweating to the next level and spend 30 minutes daily in a sauna to speed up the process.

Sharing space with a cleanse and detox expert means nothing to my dad, who believes that sickness comes and gets him. He doesn't see that his immune system is weak and that his body is full of toxins. Toxins that make his body puffy, stuffed up, creaky, in pain, on fire and that cause arthritis in his joints. His knee hurts and he is struggling to walk but will not believe that inflammation is at the cause of this pain. If only he alkalized his body and reduced the acidic causing food, he would feel his pain dissipating. The body is a very smart and powerful

315

machine, but if it is not getting optimal fuel and if it is being fed too much acidic food, then the body will be on fire. When the body is on fire, sickness sets in and so does arthritic joint pain.

When the body is dirty, it starts to break down. It seems so simple to me that we just have to clean the body. If the body is dirty, there will be pain inside. It also seems so simple to me how to clean the body. Yet the most difficult part for people is to let go of their fear of cleansing and their fear of letting their crap go. We feel safe with all the crap we carry around on the outside and the inside. We don't like to let anything go. We like to hang on. Yet this hanging on is causing us to be sick and heavy. It is time for us to LIGHTEN up, to ENLIGHTEN and release all the old baggage and crap that is holding us heavily down in a lower vibration of our reality. Lighten up, vibrate higher and have a more extraordinary life.

Another big fear for people is, "if I don't eat, I will starve", and this is the furthest from the truth, as eating lots of juices and smoothies will actually fill us up.

The first belief we have to take on is that the body is a self healing mechanism always working 24/7 for our optimal health.

The second belief is that sickness is co-created by us and our body. Our mind plays a massive role in our sickness or in our health. We create it and we can un create it.

The third belief is that if we want to heal the body, all we have to do is clean it and clean our mind. Our body will respond very quickly to this support and happily start cleaning house.

If we can believe that this is the way sickness or healing in the body works, then we are the most empowered beings ever. We can powerfully create our healing and let go of sickness and pain in our body by simply doing a JUICY cleanse for 7+ days as often as is needed.

I also suggest we continue looking within. Everything in our lives and our interactions with people is a reflection and our mirror. If we don't like something about someone, then what is it that we don't like about ourselves. If there is something about someone that annoys us, then we fix it in ourselves. If we love a character trait about another, then we witness it in our self also. It's our ride. It's our movie. It's our reality. Perhaps no one else exists and we have cast all these people into roles in our movie. Maybe when we die, we will wake up in a space ship bed on Jupiter hooked up to tubes and realize that this whole life time on earth has been one big dream, we were actively dreaming up. Perhaps it is time to get into the driver's seat of our life, take our life and our health into our hands. Perhaps it is time to be the greatest expression of our self on this planet, to fully go for our life and to have the healthiest body, mind and soul for our life journey.

WE ARE CONSCIOUS ENERGY
LIVING INSIDE A SKIN BAG
MADE OF BONES, MUSCLES & LIQUIDS
WALKING AROUND A PLANET
FLYING THROUGH OUTER SPACE
WE ARE MIRACLES
WE ARE COSMIC STARDUST
OUR LIFE MATTERS

- - ♡ - -

CHAPTER 53

AFTER LOG 2 & PETRA'S COCONUT WATER CLEANSE

Aloha my friends! As I sit here editing and spell checking this fabulous book, I am on day 7 of my coconut water cleanse. I am drinking only coconut water and spring water with the occasional juicy piece of fruit and coconut milk. I wanted to share my experience to support you further in doing your cleanse and give you the encouragement to start cleansing.

I have been travelling for the past few months and staying in very cold climates (never again as my body really does not like the cold). I was eating healthy but not the caliber of life force and juiciness I enjoy. My body and my stomach were much more acidic and out of balance. Upon returning to Bali, I had planned to do a coconut water cleanse and the universe answered my desire much faster than I had anticipated. Goddess Bali works in mysterious magical ways.

At my departure airport I purchased a bottled fruit juice and slowly sipped it. The acidity of the juice and the acidity of my stomach was too much and my body wanted the toxins out. So I started to throw up. On my return flight to Bali, I threw up 7 or more times on the plane and at my layover airport. Luckily the airplane bathrooms were available as each sensation of needing to purge came on. This of course made my 20 hour return trip feel so much longer. There are no accidents and I did declare to the universe that I wanted to cleanse and so I got as I asked for. I watch the signs from the universe and know I am taken care of. So I loved myself through the process, knew I was ok and that this was ultimately all for my highest good.

I arrived to Bali completely purged and ready to move right into my coconut water and spring water cleanse. Because my body had already purged out a lot of my stomach acid and toxins, it was easier to transition to just drinking water. If I started my cleanse after eating a big meal, the onboarding experience would be much tougher. Since my body hadn't eaten for over 24 hours and I had already gone through the nausea experience, I was already over the initial cleansing hump.

I am on day 7 and I feel great. At times I do feel hungry and when I do, I suck back gulps of coconut water and the hunger pangs go away. I drink at least 4 coconuts every day, sometimes more. I drink spring water and have a few pieces of watermelon to help me through the hungry times. I sip on coconut milk in the evening, as the fat helps fill me up. A few days ago I ate a few raw crackers. Since I have done so much cleansing in my life, I don't feel I need to be super strict with myself. If I wanted to super cleanse, I would stay home, sleep a lot more and drink only water for my 7 days.

My energy levels are great. My body feels great. I do have the desire to sleep more and I give my body the time to rest. My tongue is extra white as the toxins are showing up on my tongue, showing me that I want to keep going to cleanse it further. When I feel hungry throughout my day, I drink another coconut. I will transition to a juice cleanse to follow this and then eat mainly raw food for the rest of the month. I am choosing to youthen, regenerate my body, clean out my cells (which store my toxins) and give my body a reboot.

Cleansing is not easy, yet it is not difficult either. It is mainly in the mind that we desire to eat and feel a lack when we are not. I am sitting here dreaming about all the yummy restaurants and this makes me feel hungry. I just keep saying to myself, all in good time. I will be eating soon, but for now I am healing my body. My health is my most important asset, so I have the motivation to keep my cleanse going.

What is your motivation? Do you want to live a longer, healthier, happier, freer life?

If so, then its time to join me in the cleansing world and start your JUICY cleanse today. I am right here with you, holding your hand all the way. You can do this. Your life and your health depend on you taking charge. Don't wait until you are sick, have pain or look old. Cleansing is preventative medicine to live a long healthy vibrant life.

The scariest place any of us can be is hearing that we are sick, have cancer or are going to die. Or hearing that our loved ones are diagnosed this way. It does not have to be like this. We do not have to wait till we get sick or are dying to make a change, we can make a change right now. It is my intention that this book and my online JUICY cleanse 7 day video program help you take your health into your hands RIGHT NOW!

I hope you feel much more confident and equipped to cleanse your body and heal yourself after reading this book. You are powerful and your body is a self healing miraculous machine that is healing you in every moment. Just get out of it's way. Stop eating the crap. Stop eating solid food for a few days and flush out your system. Let go of all that is no longer serving you and get rid of the years of built up toxins that are living in your cells, tissues, organs and blood stream.

It is easy for you to be healthy, energized, vibrant, youthful and live for a long time. It is up to you. Are you willing to say YES to yourself and to your new happier and freer life?

Are you willing to say YES to you?...

IT'S TIME TO JUICY CLEANSE!!!
LET'S DO THIS
SAY YES
I GOT YOUR BACK!

- - ♡ - -

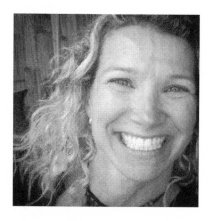

Petra EatJuicy, is a Super Hero Level Holistic Health Coach, Detox Expert, Author, Raw Food Chef, Theta Healing Practitioner, Yogini & Juicy Lifestyle Activist. She travels the world speaking, teaching and coaching about natural eating, self healing, mindfulness, self love and personal empowerment. She and her team tour the world empowering people, to take their health into their own hands by joining Green Smoothie Gangster Health Challenge.
She lives in Bali, Maui, Canada & Czech Republic.

Check out her amazing online coaching programs to reverse cancer, heal your gut, lose weight without counting calories and live your most vibrant self expressed life.

www.EatJuicy.com
www.GreenSmoothieGangster.com

www.Facebook.com/PetraEatJuicy
www.Youtube.com/PetraEatJuicy
www.Instagram.com/PetraEatJuicy

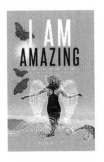

I Am Amazing

A No-Nonsense Self Love Guide To Remember Your Greatness & Rock Out Your Life! Empower Yourself, Feel Happier, Heal Your Body & Become Your Own Best Friend

- Petra EatJuicy, Green Smoothie Gangster

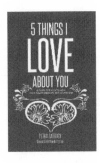

5 Things I Love About You

A Game For You To Heal Your Relationships With Everyone

- Petra EatJuicy, Green Smoothie Gangster

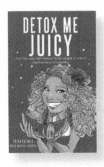

Detox Me Juicy

A 7 Day Juicy Food Cleanse To Lose Weight, Youthen & Heal Your Body Of Everything

- Petra EatJuicy, Green Smoothie Gangster

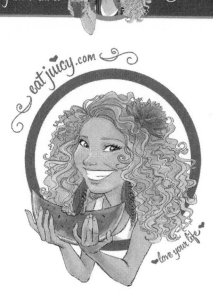

eat juicy.com

love your life

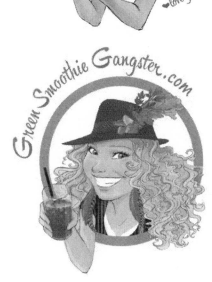

Green Smoothie Gangster.com